Frequently Asked Questions on Sex

Frequently Asked Questions on Sex

Dr. Vijai Rikh
Senior Sex Therapist and Consultant
Delhi

PEEPEE
PUBLISHERS and DISTRIBUTORS (P) LTD.

Frequently Asked Questions on Sex

Published by
Pawaninder P. Vij
Peepee Publishers and Distributors (P) Ltd.

7/31, Ansari Road, Daryaganj,
New Delhi 110002 (India)
Ph: 55195868, 9811156083
e-mail: peepee160@yahoo.co.in
e-mail: peepee160@rediffmail.co.in

First Edition: **2004**

ISBN 81-88867-08-X

Printed at
Lordson, C-5/19, Rana Pratap Bagh, Delhi-110 007

To

My Grand Children

Abhishek, Pallavi, Abhilasha, Mayank

I

Dedicate this book

with love and affection

PREFACE

The aim of this book is to replace ignorance with knowledge and for achieving this goal it is written to answer questions that crop up in the minds of young and old alike.

I am sure this book would enlighten every one and provide latest information especially to those who are abysmally ignorant about 'Sex' and 'Sexuality'.

Dr. Rikh

ACKNOWLEDGEMENT

I am really indebted to my sons Rajiv Rikh and Sanjiv Rikh (presently in U.S.) and daughter–in–laws Saroj Bala Rikh and Pratibha Rikh for their encouragement, inspiration and moral support to complete this book.

Lastly I acknowledge my gratitude to my assistant Shiv Kumar Sharma for his last minute corrections and typing the manuscript in a very short span of time enabling me to handover the same to my publisher Pawaninder P. Vij at my earliest.

Dr. Rikh

Dear Readers

This book contains a wide spectrum of questions, the answers of which you wanted to know from your parents or teachers but due to natural shyness fail to do so resulting in abysmal ignorance and wrong notions.

Here you would find their correct answers, which would not only increase your knowledge about 'Sex' and 'Sexuality' but also enable you to face the realities of life in a much better way than before.

But still if you have any query or problem you can write me on the address given below:

Dr. Rikh
C-2B/69A, Janakpuri,
New Delhi – 110058.

Email: drrikh@eth.net
Visit us at: www.indiansexologist.com

Delaying the Climax

Q. A friend of mine wants to know if there is any way in which he can delay his climax as he ejaculates after 60 or seventy strokes and his wife gets no satisfaction.
He said he read once in one of the magazines about some kind of ointment, which is applied to the head of the organ to delay the climax. He went to a chemist and told him he would like some ointment that delay his climax and the chemist gave him did not help a bit.

Ans. If your friend does not ejaculate until 60 or 70 strokes after intromission, he is completely adequate in his staying power. The solution to this problem probably should be sought elsewhere than in delaying ejaculation. What your friend should pay more attention to is learning to stimulate his wife sufficiently in fore-play so that she can be brought to climax earlier. Perhaps the wife may be too tardy in her responses.

Vaginal Relaxation

Q. My husband apparently knows much less about sex, believes that I am unfaithful to him. He is convinced that, because my vagina seems "loose," I have had relations with other men. Is there any way I can convince him he is wrong?
What causes this condition of relaxation and what can be done to correct it?

Ans. Your husband apparently knows much less about sex than he thinks he does. There is absolutely no way he could know that you had relations with another merely from the "looseness" of the vagina. Even a doctor would have difficulty in establishing this.

The looseness you speak of may come from a result of the fluids, which are released by the vaginal glands under sexual excitement. An alum solution is sometimes helpful in alleviating too great lubrication but it should not be too strong.

It is also possible that there is a relaxation of the muscles, which needs correction, on advice of a gynecologist.

Let him know that, in a doctor's opinion he is completely wrong in trying to make judgments without understanding enough about sex anatomy.

Relaxed Vagina

Q. Can you give me some information on what to do about a relaxed vagina? I am 36 year old and I seem to have loss all control. When I have intercourse, my vagina is more relaxed than it should be, which makes it difficult for my husband to enjoy our relations. Is there anything that can be done?

Ans. You do not give us any information as to whether or not you have children. If you have and the vagina was torn, and not repaired at the time of childbirth, the only thing to do is to have the vagina repaired. This is called a vaginal plastic operation.

Of course, as you get older, normal tissue firmness decreases. This makes you feel now at 36, that your vagina is more relaxed. If the vagina is not torn, one can develop the muscles of the vagina simply by contracting them, and squeezing as hard as one can. This is the same feeling that you have when you are attempting to prevent urination. The procedure is to contract the muscles, hold them as long as possible, and then release them, and repeat this exercise 10 or 12 times, one right after the other, and do the whole exercise 5 to 8 times a day. In the course of a month or 6 weeks, a considerable capacity to contract the vagina may be developed.

Genital Size

Q. I am 26 year old and married. I believe that my sexual organ is too small and would like it to be much larger. When I have coitus with my wife I find that I am much smaller than she is and do not get the proper sensation. Please advise me the best way that I can develop a larger sexual organ. It is just five inches long when tumescent.

Also, my wife's breasts are very small and we would both like to find a way to make them larger. Is there any medicine that would solve our problem? Is there any exercise plan that would solve our problem? What about surgery (if possible we would like to have this done)? Who would we see, what does it usually cost and how successful is surgery? What about the ointments that are advertised? In general can her breasts be greatly increased in size and what would be your best suggestion?

Ans. There is no need for you to be concerned about your organ. Your dimensions are entirely adequate. Any lack of satisfaction you may have is definitely not caused by genital size.

There is no safe method of increasing the size of your genital, and trying to do so is not only doubtful but will cause you to neglect your real problem, which may come from too little knowledge about sex techniques.

A gynecologist should examine your wife. Perhaps there is a condition (poor muscle tone, etc.), which can be corrected without too much difficulty.

Medicine or exercise cannot make your wife's breasts

larger unless she suffers from a lack of female hormone. Then an endocrinologist should treat her. Plastic surgery is possible, but it is very expensive, and it is not successful in many cases because doctors have not succeeded in discovering a material, which can be implanted in the breast safely and without hardening or lumping.

The best thing for your wife and you would be to realize that sex happiness does not depend either on the size of genitals or breasts, but upon the quality of your love for each other and your mutual concern to discover the ways of making each other happy.

Penis Length

Q. When having sexual intercourse is it necessary for the male organ to extend the full length of a woman's vagina in order for her to reach full satisfaction? In other words, if the man's penis is too small in relation to the woman, is it possible to satisfy her?

Ans. It is not at all necessary for a penis to be long enough to reach the very end of the vagina in order to give a woman complete sexual satisfaction. The sensory organs are at the entrance to the vagina, and in the clitoris, which is about an inch and half above the entrance to the vagina. The petting, caressing, consideration, and loving attention which a man gives to a woman is far more important than size of his penis. If husband and wife will open up channels of communication, and if the two are willing to cooperate to obtain a more satisfactory and mutual sexual relationship, they can usually overcome any such problem.

Enlarging Penis

Q. I am suffering from a complex because my penis is too small. I want to know where I can buy an apparatus to enlarge my organ. I have heard of one type that works by suction.

Ans. Any of the so-called suction apparatuses that are supposed to enlarge the penis actually do not do so. The danger is that they bring about a change in the internal structure of the penis, which may be very seriously harmful. I can only advise very strongly against the use of any such apparatus.

Vaginal Depth

Q. What I have read about the size of vagina has left me confused. I have seen the figure of the average depth given by experts as about three inches. In that case, how is it possible to accommodate even the average male organ, which is perhaps double that length?

Ans. Measured from the hymen, the average depth of the vagina is 3 to 3 and 1/2 inches. When you include the Vulva, or external female parts, you find that the average length of the coital passage is close to 6 inches. You must also remember that the vagina is a highly elastic organ and hence expands to accommodate a penis of any size. Were this not so, childbirth would be impossible.

Breast Stimulation

Q. I have heard that stimulation of the female breast is Important during marital relations and I would

like to know exactly what role the female breast has in marital relations and how important this role is. What are the Average dimensions of the female breast and nipples?

Ans. The breasts are closely allied with the entire sexual system. Stimulation of them pervious to intercourse and during coitus usually gives a woman a gratifying feeling, and in may cases, a sense of intense sexual excitation. The nipples erect and it is but natural that numerous psychological changes occur during stimulation. The average dimensions of the breasts and nipples of the human female have not been established. It must be remembered that even in one individual the breasts will vary in size at different ages and under different physical conditions. Lactation also changes shape and size.

Oral-Genital Contacts

Q. **I know there are men and women who occasionally engage in oral relations as an extra stimulus to normal sexual intercourse with the opposite sex. Does doing this indicate a homosexual disposition? At what ages are these acts most craved?**

Ans. When these sexual acts are indulged in between members of the opposite sex they indicate heterosexual feelings, not homosexual. They are fairly common practices performed by married couples—especially among the better educated. Mouth genital contacts are also to be widely observed between males and females of the lower mammals.

Unfortunately, there is no data available concerning at which ages the cravings are most strong. Certainly the behavior has been more prevalent among our younger generation.

Oral Sex

Q. I am 28 years old and considered a very beautiful woman. I have been married twice before and I am now engaged to a man of 43. Our problem is that he refuses to indulge in oral-genital relations, which I find necessary as foreplay in order to attain a climax.

We are very much in love. I want to know if it is wrong for me to want him to do this. I don't want to encourage him to do anything bad.

Ans. Oral-genital contacts are far more common than was ordinarily believed prior to the Kinsey report. As to whether or not it is wrong, that is a private matter. Leading marriage and religious counselors believe that any form or stimulation that is mutually desired and does not involve cruelty is appropriate in marriage. Perhaps discussion with a marriage counselor would be worthwhile so that this and other problems can be worked out.

Coitus in Menstruation

Q. Most of the women with whom I have discussed the problem tell me that, although they sometimes have desire for sex relations during their menstrual period, they refrain because of the fear of harm. Is sex during menses injurious to health and objectionable in other ways?

Ans. Sexual intercourse during menstruation is known to have been practiced since the beginning of recorded history. Since the very early centuries of the present era, the most highly recognized physicians have stated that sexual intercourse during menstruation is not unhygienic and not unhealthy. This is also the view prevailing among medical authorities today.

Whether or not intercourse is practiced at this time, is a matter of preference of individuals.

Length of Coitus

Q. During the past six years disharmony between my husband and me has increased because he has been unable to prolong the sex act. He reaches a climax in about three minutes. In all our marital relations in a month, I usually have only one climax. Isn't there something wrong in his reaching a climax in so quick a time? How long should normal intercourse take?

Ans. There are a great many variations in the length of intercourse for different men. There may also be great variations in time for any one individual on different occasions because of a number of factors (sex tension, frequency of coitus, etc.).

Most studies have established that the average time after intromission and active movements have begun is about two minutes. Thus your husband prolongs his climax somewhat longer than does the average male. What is probably needed in your sex relations is a longer period of foreplay and erotic stimulation prior to intromission.

Many men fail to realize how necessary is such preparation of the wife, who generally takes longer to be completely aroused and ready for the sex act. As has often been said, the wife has to be wooed again before every marital act.

Perhaps also you require a different type of stimulation during coitus in order to achieve climax more quickly. A greater knowledge of marital techniques by both you and your husband would undoubtedly result in greater mutual satisfaction

---

Excessive Masturbation

Q. Sometimes during the discussion of case histories, the term "excessive masturbation: is mentioned. How often is considered excessive?

Ans. The average frequency of masturbation is probably 2 times a week in a young unmarried man. But there really is no exact figure that we can use to distinguish between normal and excessive masturbation. Once a month might be enough for one individual and once a day might not be too much for another.

Masturbation would be considered excessive only when it becomes a compulsive type of behavior where the individual simply cannot get it off his mind and is never free from the feeling or the urge to indulge in it. Besides, masturbation is self-limiting. Before "excess," there is simply no more erection possible.

Lack of Tumescence

Q. I am 34 years old and every time that I proceed with the sexual act, I find that erection of the organ does not take place. I will appreciate advice or the prescription of some efficient remedy.

Ans. No doctor could prescribe an efficient remedy for your condition without having a chance to examine you personally. Therefore the wisest thing you could do is to consult a sexologist personally.

He could tell you, after proper tests, whether there is any physical cause of your condition. If so, he might prescribe a remedy.

However, in most cases lack of erection comes from fear, lack of confidence, or some kind of emotional anxiety. If this is true in your case, you would need psychological help to give you a feeling of confidence. Once you get this confidence you may find that your difficulty has completely disappeared. By all means see a doctor.

Anesthetic Ejaculation

Q. Is there anything that can be done for my husband? He has no trouble attaining an erection but when he reaches an orgasm there is no feeling and he ends up discouraged. He is 33 years old. I very seldom reach a climax, so could that have any effect on the way he feels?

Ans. Your husband's condition is known as anesthetic ejaculation. The cause of this is not definitely known. There may be a physical cause, or a number of such causes, but it has been found that a large number of such cases have a psychological basis. For some reason a man may, without being at all aware of it, lose his appreciation of the sensations of the orgasm. Many victims of this condition have been helped by psychotherapy.

Your husband's condition should not be affected by your lack of climax.

Artificial Organ

Q. I am 41 years old and I have been married fifteen years. My problem is that I have an immediate climax as soon as coitus begins. Since my wife now refuses to have marital relations, I decided to ask my physician for an artificial rubber organ that my wife might use. However, when I reached the doctor's office, I became embarrassed because he refused to help me in direction. Where could I find a physician who could prescribe such an artificial organ?

Ans. No doctor will prescribe an artificial rubber penis because there are none such on the legitimate market, and doctors do not prescribe or recommend them because they are of no value and may do harm.

It would be unwise for you to think that an artificial organ would solve your problem in any way. You are still both very young and all your efforts should be directed to trying to work out satisfactory sex relations with each other.

It is clear that both of you need some kind of help and you should try to seek it from a sexologist competent in this field or from a marriage counselor. You should have a sexologist examine you first to find out if there is a physical basis for your quick ejaculation. Some men have found it helpful to apply a local anesthetic cream to the glans penis from half an hour to several hours before coitus. This mild anesthetic would desensitize the organ and enable you to impart sufficient number of strokes. However nowadays apart from medicines some exercises as 'Start & Stop Technique' really work and produce very satisfying results.

Homosexuality

Q. I am 32 years old and physically well developed. Since I was small my sexual desires have been toward men only. I would like to be married but fear that I could not make a woman happy. On two different occasions I have been with a woman but did not feel sex desire. I wish to change my feelings toward women. You know many cases like mine. I hope that you will help me.

Ans. Many men who are homosexuals are not potent with women. It is very difficult for a homosexual to change his sexual desires and direct them toward women. If the condition can be corrected at all, it requires expert psychiatric help. Certainly marriage should not be undertaken before you seek such help. It would be fair neither to you nor the woman involved.

Since you desire to change you should try to get help, although it is costly. It may help you to be happier, either by changing your sex orientation or by accepting your condition if it cannot be changed.

Homosexual Acceptance

Q. Are there any countries where homosexuality is permitted? I know that in almost every state in the U.S. a man can be sent to jail for performing homosexual acts.

Ans. There is no country where homosexuals are fully accepted by the general population. However, they are fairly well tolerated in Denmark and Holland. So long as they do nothing to involve younger individuals, little is done by the way of persecution or punishment in these 2 countries. In many states private acts between adults are not punished in practice, but acts done in public or involving youngsters are penalized.

Feeling Orgasm

Q. How can the male partner tell if the female has reached orgasm? It seems possible that a woman could pretend to reach orgasm.

Ans. The female has the same convulsive contractions of the pelvic muscles as occurs in the male when he reaches a climax in intercourse. There is the same deep spasmodic breathing. Some women can simulate this so effectively that a man cannot be sure whether or not they have actually reached orgasm.

Simultaneous Orgasm

Q. I have been married for 6 years. My wife and I can't reach orgasm at the same time. The problem arises because I can't make good contact with the clitoris. Is there a position we can use that will help us?

Ans. You are undoubtedly over-emphasizing the necessity or desirability of attempting to achieve orgasm at the same time. The important thing is that both of you should achieve orgasm.

With a little experimentation and imagination on your part, you should be able to get into a position, which is easy and comfortable. By doing this you can bring your wife along to the point of orgasm so that, if you do wish to have the experience of attaining it together, you may be able to achieve it.

Clitoral Stimulation

Q. I used to manipulate my wife's clitoris for a long time before engaging in the sex act. Is it wrong or right? My wife had taught me that she preferred this form of stimulation to coitus itself.

Ans. In speaking of clitoral manipulation you asked "Is it wrong or right?" If you speak of right or wrong in a moral sense, no problem of ethics is involved where marital practices are agreeable to both husband and wife.

Physically, the practice is natural and harmless, and as a matter of fact far more important in bringing about satisfaction for the female than is generally realized.

The requirements of women (for sexual satisfaction) differ vastly from the requirements of men. You should be guided by your wife's desires in this instance. Of course, your wife should also make certain that you also obtain satisfaction.

Sexual Response

Q. Does the physical size of the wife or husband have any bearing on sexual satisfaction? I have seen big women and little men and big men and little women as partners and I was wondering if the physical size has any bearing on sexual union. Does a woman who is a virgin at the time of marriage respond to sexual feeling as freely as a girl who has been sexually free before marriage? My wife was 20 years old at marriage and was a virgin. She responds very well as a sex partner.

Ans. Physical dimension are not related to the ability to achieve marital satisfaction. In the first place, genital size is not related to height and weight. Secondly, marital gratification is a product of many factors. The most important is the love and total relationship of the partners.

Just to what extent any woman responds to sexual intercourse depends on the individual woman. No general statement is possible. Many so-called "loose" women are actually frigid. Many virgins respond strongly, just as your wife did.

Curved Organ

Q. I am 27 years old and am unmarried. As early as I can remember my organ has been crooked (it slants to the left). I am very sensitive about this and would like to know what measures I can take to straighten it, if any at all. I don't know if this was

caused by masturbation or if I was simply born this way. Perhaps you can tell me what might have caused this and what remedies I can take to correct it.

Ans. The bent, curved or arched penis is quite common. It is not caused by the practice of self-gratification. The reason is to be found in the hollow bodies of the penis.

These hollow bodies are not equalized in capacity. Therefore, when they are filled with blood the erect organ tends to curve. Pronounced arching is often a congenital trait.

The condition generally follows a heredity pattern and usually does not in any way affect sexual functioning. Pills and other "remedies" that one may take naturally are ineffective. A large number of your fellow men have the same condition and the population of the world continues to increase.

Sensitiveness on your part only causes you to suffer. Ignore the condition and you will find no interference with your sex gratification. If it gets worse, see an urologist.

Nymphomania

Q. I am 32 years old and my wife is 26. My wife's sexual demands are so great that it is impossible for me to satisfy her. We have sexual intercourse every morning and night, 3 or 4 times daily. Furthermore, I have been informed that my wife has been seeking satisfaction with other men. And to make the problem even worse, her sex desires are becoming more and more intense instead of less.

I have heard about nymphomania. What is it and what causes it? What sort of specialist should we go to?

Ans. Nymphomania means insatiable sex desire.

The cause is generally psychological, but occasionally, this is brought on by some vaginal irritation or an irritation around the clitoris. If, for instance, this tiny organ has a fold of skin over it and there are lumps of smegma secretions underneath causing continual irritation, it may bring about almost an insatiable sexual desire.

The only suggestion we can make is that you have your wife consult a gynecologist to rule out any possible physical causes. If there is none, she should consult a psychiatrist.

Prolonging Relations

Q. My wife and I have intercourse every night and the longer we can keep it up the better we like it. The problem is that it takes me a very long time to reach orgasm but my wife gets through very quickly. I was wondering if my wife could delay orgasm the way men sometimes do by using some Xylocaine Ointment on her sex organs. Before we try it we want to know if it is harmful.

Ans. Your wife might try a little of the Xylocaine Ointment just around the entrance of the vagina and just inside of the vagina and also put some on the clitoris. This might make it possible for her to prolong intercourse also. It is not considered harmful.

Coitus Reservatus

Q. I am writing this because I disagree with your stand on coitus reservatus. You constantly warn to of the dangers of this practice. (In coitus reservatus

the male ends intercourse without ejaculation occurring at all.)

I have practiced reservatus on a steadily increasing scale, ever since boyhood, to a degree of quantity and quality that taxes even my own imagination and belief. I am 49 years of age and in perfect health, never having been ill, except by accident, a day of my life.

Ans. You must understand first of all that each case of health or disease is a law unto itself. That which might do your neighbor irreparable damage might not harm you at all. It is for this reason that our answers have to be general and do not necessarily apply to all individuals.

Undoubtedly many persons such as you have practiced coitus reservatus without any ill effects whatsoever. The famous Oneida Community, which practiced complete suppression of ejaculation, was supposed to have been certified as medically healthy.

However, we have made it a practice to warn our readers against reservatus because a number of urologists are of the opinion that suppression of ejaculation over a long period of time may have very harmful effects on the prostate gland. They feel that the congestion in the gland, which is brought about by sexual arousal, is harmful if it does not lead to adequate emptying of the gland. When prostatic fluid is not completely discharged, it undergoes changes, which often create inflammation and deterioration of the healthy tissue.

Since there is a great possibility that harm may ensure from this practice, we have warned our readers against it. This of course does not mean that in your particular case any harm has been done. Sexual response is a very individual one and varies greatly from person to person.

Anal Relations

Q. I am a happily married woman. Recently, my husband and I had perverted intercourse; that is, we had intercourse anally rather than vaginally. We liked this new experience, but we have not done it again. I would like to know if it is harmful in any way.

Ans. Anal intercourse is sometimes used as a method of intercourse where pregnancy is undesired, or as a variation in relations. If it is not painful and does not cause you any discomfort or distress, it is essentially harmless. However, there is always a slight possibility of a urethral infection from some of the organism in the bowel, but aside from this it should do no harm. However, you should understand that this type of intercourse is considered immoral by most religions and even illegal by some state laws.

Clitoris

Q. I think that quite a few men (and maybe some women) do not understand and appreciate the function of the clitoris. Would you please write about that "organ?"

Ans. The clitoris is located toward the front or top of a woman's external genitals. The head of the clitoris, about the size of a small pea, is often visible or can be seen by gently pushing up the skin covering it. The size and appearance of the clitoris vary among women. Most of it is inside and not visible.

As a woman becomes sexually aroused, the clitoris pulls back against the pubic bone and the labia swell so that the head is protected from direct touch. Shortly after orgasm, the clitoris resumes its unstimulated position.

Contrary to popular myth, the head of the clitoris is not some type of "magic button" for all women and, in fact, direct stimulation is uncomfortable or even painful for some. A touch that contributes to sexual responsiveness for one woman can be painful to another woman—an example of why communication between sexual partners is necessary.

G-Spot

Q. I am 54 years old and up until recently have never heard of the trigger or "G" spot in a woman. There was even a lengthy story in Playboy, which I just read. Truthfully, is there such a thing, and, if so, where?

Ans. There has been considerable debate over the existence of the G spot or Grafenberg spot, named for Ernest Grafenberg, the German gynecologist who first described it. The results of studies on the G spot vary widely. Some researchers have found no evidence of it, while other report finding a highly sensitive spot on the vaginal wall of some women that has the characteristics of the G spot.

The G spot is said to be a small mass of tissue (the size and shape of a small bean) about 2 inches inside the vaginal opening on the front wall of the vagina (the side toward the belly button). This area is reputed to be highly sensitive to sexual stimulation, during which the area becomes larger, about the size of a dime.

Many experts feel more research is necessary before the existence of the G spot can be established, but there is no question many women notice that some areas of the vagina are more sensitive to erotic touch than others.

Fate of Semen

Q. I am 65. After intercourse, what happens to the semen that remains in my body? Is that dangerous? Should I douche? This has troubled me for a long time.

Ans. The semen does not stay in your body. It gradually runs out of the vagina after intercourse. A healthy vagina cleans itself naturally, as secretions work their way to the external genitals. This means that carefully washing and rinsing the folds of the external genitals each day is all the cleaning most women need.

Female Internal Genitalia

Q. Sir, I want to know about the female's reproductive system and the various functions each organ performs?

Ans. Most of the female's reproductive system is inside her body. The two **ovaries**, which produce eggs and hormones, are each about the size of a grape (approximately 1 inch by ½ inch). At birth, each ovary contains approximately 200,000 immature eggs. Each egg is surrounded by a thin tissue envelope called a **follicle.** Each ovary is attached to one end of an **ovarian ligament** (a band of fibrous tissue). The other end of each ligament is attached to the uterus.

One common misconception is that the ovaries are also attached to the Fallopian tubes (named for the Italian anatomist who first described them), since an egg released by an ovary must travel through one of the Fallopian tubes to reach the uterus. Indeed, one end of each Fallopian tube (about 4 inches long and about as big around as a piece of spaghetti) is attached to the top area of the uterus, but the other end simply dangles near an ovary. The outer ends are formed somewhat like a funnel-shaped flower with fringelike extensions called fimbria. When an egg is released from an ovary the fimbria wave about, surround the ovary, and draw the egg into the Fallopian tube near that ovary. The inside of each Fallopian tube is lined with cilia, tiny hair like structures that also move. Conception occurs when an egg and sperm meet inside one of the Fallopian tubes, which is where the embryo begins to grow.

The uterus (also called the womb) is about the size and shape of a pear (about 3 inches long and 2 inches wide) but much flatter. It is made of muscle (the outer layer called the myometrium) and has a special inner lining (the endometrium), which first builds up and then leaves the body as menstrual flow in each reproductive cycle when conception does not occur. If conception does occur, the fertilized egg travels through a Fallopian tube into the uterus, where it implants in the endometrium and uses the nutrients of the lining for the early stages of embryonic development. It is quite remarkable that the small uterus can expand over the course of nine months to accommodate a full-size newborn.

The bottom part of the uterus is called the cervix (Latin for "neck"). The cervix is connected to and protrudes into the upper end of the vagina. In the center of the cervix is a small hole, the os ("mouth" in Latin), through which menstrual flow passes from the uterus to the vagina. It is also through the os that sperm must swim from the vagina into the uterus and then into the Fallopian tubes to meet an egg. During labor, the os greatly enlarges (dilates) for passage of the newborn.

The vagina is a small tube (about 3 to 4 inches long) made of muscle and covered on the inside walls with a mucous surface similar to the lining of the mouth;

this surface produces vaginal lubrication. Unless a woman is sexually aroused, the sides of the vagina touch each other. When a woman becomes sexually aroused the walls of the vagina produce a slippery liquid and balloon opens so that a penis will fit inside. It can open even further to permit passage of a fully-grown newborn.

Vaginal Discharge

Q. I am 20-year-old woman who occasionally has a white jellylike vaginal discharge. The texture is very much like gelatin. It is not the usual yellow or white creamy discharge. This occurs about once every two months. What is this? Is it anything to be alarmed about?

Ans. What you have noticed is probably either normal cervical mucus or vaginal lubricating fluid. If you have no other symptoms (such as vaginal itching, soreness, or pain), the changes you've seen probably are normal. Ask about this during your next annual pelvic exam so that physician can check the condition of your cervix or take samples of secretions for analysis.

The appearance and texture of vaginal secretions vary throughout each monthly reproductive cycle as conditions inside the vagina respond to changes in hormonal levels. This is especially true of the mucus secreted by the cervix.

Cervical mucus usually appears in greater quantities midcycle, around the time the egg is released, and color and texture then differ from vaginal secretions during the rest of the month. The special mucus facilitates the journey of the sperm through the cervix into the uterus. In addition, the lubricating fluid produced by the vagina during sexual arousal also looks different from other vaginal secretions.

Public Hair

Q. Why is the hair around the genitals called public when in a sense it is very private?

Ans. The hair in question is called pubic, not public. Dictionaries note that the phrase "pubic hair" is related to both the pubic bone (which is under the hair) and puberty (the time of development when the hair first appears on the genitals.)

Penile Curves

Q. I am 19 years old. My problem is that when I have an erection, my penis gets a slight curve in it and it can be very embarrassing when I get into sexual situations. I was wondering if there is a special physician I could see for this problem or a special procedure that can be done to correct my problem.

Ans. It is not unusual for an erect penis to have a slight curve. Asked about the angle and shape of their penis, about 20 percent of men said it points straight out from the body when erect, 5 percent said it points down, and the rest said it points upward. Some reported that the angle became more downward as they got older. More than half of men said their erect penises are centered in relation to their bodies, about 30 percent said the penis aims to the left, and about 6 percent reported that it aims to the right. However, if the curve is severe enough to make sexual penetration difficult or if having an erection is painful, you should consult a urologist.

A few men do have more severe curves. Some are born with penile structural problems, such as a short urethra that can cause the penis to severely bend (called chordee). A different type of penile curve that suddenly appears much later in life can be a symptom of Peyronie's disease.

Short Frenulum

Q. As a very much younger man I tore my "G" string and I've wondered since exactly what it was that I tore. The short membrane, or cord, that holds the foreskin forward. Would you give me the anatomical nomenclature of this important presence?

Ans. From your description it sounds as though the name you're looking for is *frenulum preputii*, the fold of skin (frenulum) that passes from under the glans of the penis to the skin covering the penis shaft.

The human body has many such folds of skin. (There is one between the undersurface of the tongue and the bottom of the mouth and another beneath the upper lip, between the lip and gum.) Tearing the frenulum you refer to is not unusual.

Such a tear may produce a great deal of blood, but it usually heals spontaneously. These tears require surgery only if any scar tissue that forms hinders movement of the penile skin or causes discomfort. Most men find this particular frenulum especially sensitive to erotic touching.

Tight Foreskin

Q. As an uncircumcised male, I've found that I have pain during intercourse, occurring at the first stage of penetration. Also, I'm unable to pull back my foreskin. I'm sure these two conditions are interrelated. Is circumcision the answer?

Ans. Circumcision may not be necessary. Check with a physician, preferably a urologist, to determine why your foreskin is not moving freely and if this is related to your pain during intercourse. If the problem is an infection, antibiotics may correct the problem. Or the foreskin opening can sometimes be surgically enlarged so that it will more easily permit retraction.

Unequal Level of Testicles

Q. Is it normal for one testicle to hang lower in the scrotum than the other testicle? The right one is almost always near the base of the penis while the left one is always lower, touching the bottom of the scrotum. Is this normal for all males?

Ans. Yes. This helps keep the testicles from being squeezed when a man's legs are together. In most men, the left testicle is lower than the right testicle. In left-handed men, the opposite is often true.

Removal of Testicles

Q. If a man has been castrated, can he ever again be sexually active? What actually happens to the body in such a case?

Ans. Research has shown that a few men can have erections and sexual relationships following castration (surgical removal of the testicles). But they would not be capable of impregnating a woman because sperm are produced only in the testicles. And because the testicles produce testosterone, the man's body would gradually show the effects of the lack of this hormone (facial hair growth would slow, for example) unless it was replaced by taking synthetic hormones.

Composition of Semen

Q. I would like to know the breakdown of semen. That is, of just what is it composed, the chemical composition, by percentage perhaps?

Ans. The chemicals in human semen vary somewhat, depending on the man's diet, health, and frequency of ejaculation, but the average ejaculate chemically consists mostly of protein, citric acid, fructose (a complex sugar), sodium, and chloride.

There are smaller amounts of ammonia, ascorbic acid, acid phosphatase, calcium, carbon dioxide, cholesterol, prostanglandins; creatine, other minerals, and numerous other chemicals.

Prostrate Gland

Q. I am a 70-year-old male. I hear more and more about cancer of the prostate gland. Where is the prostate and what is its function?

Ans. The prostate is shaped something like a small doughnut surrounding the first inch of the urethra nearest the bladder. During puberty the increase in testosterone stimulates the prostate to grow to its adult size, which is approximately an inch thick and 1.5 inches across. The prostate makes a fluid that mixes with the sperm and fluids from other male reproductive organs. These fluids come out of the male urethra and are called the ejaculate or semen. About one-third of the ejaculatory fluid is from the prostate. Researchers think the prostatic fluid, which is alkaline, plays a role in reproduction by reducing the high acidity of vaginal secretions. Sperm are not as motile (do not actively swim forward) in an acidic environment as in one that is more chemically neutral.

Even though scientists do not think the prostate plays an active role in the hormonal system, it is certainly affected by changes in other organs and hormone levels. For example, the prostate will decrease in size if testosterone levels drop or estrogen levels rise.

The prostate, the opening of the bladder, and the tubes that carry sperm and other fluids to where they mix for ejaculation are located at the inner end of the urethra. The prostate can be felt through the wall of the rectum, especially if it is enlarged for any reason. One symptom of an enlarged prostate is difficult urination (a swollen prostate gland may squeeze around the urethra and slow or block the flow of urine).

A physical examination that includes a manual examination of the prostate every year after the age of forty is important to detect any changes in the prostate gland early.

Penis Size

Q. I am 22 years old and have a problem that I am sure many other men have. The size of my penis is very small, in the flaccid State and when erect. I want know if there is any medical treatment (such as hormones or surgery or vacuum pump or some creams or some kind of exercises) to correct this defect. I am very much desperate. Therefore please reply at your earliest.

Ans. No exercise, pills, creams, pumps, vitamins, injections, or any other of the hundreds of products or services advertised at the back of magazines or through direct mail—will increase the size of the adult penis. What's more, some of these products can have a harmful effect. Pump devices, for instance, have been known to damage fragile erecti tissue.

The vast majority of men measure within the average genital size range and have a penis that is approximately 5 to 7 inches long when erect, a length that is more than adequate for sexual functioning. Actual difficulties with sexual functioning or reproduction, in fact, rarely occur unless the erect penis is less than 2 inches long. In general, at erection smaller flaccid penises lengthen by a greater percentage than do larger penises. In other words, the size of a penis when it is flaccid does not predict what its size will be when erect.

From what they describe, nearly all the men who write about this worry are well within the normal size range, yet they are convinced that their penises are too small for a satisfying sexual life. Some judge themselves against the genitals depicted in erotic films and magazines, where men are usually hired precisely because they have larger-than-average penises.

Many men assume—just as women do about breasts—that the opposite sex prefers a large penis. In one study, when men were asked to list what they thought women find sexually attractive, they gave very high priority to large genitals. But the woman surveyed preferred firm muscle tone, well-groomed hair, a clear complexion, and white teeth.

Penis size is no more a measure of manhood, sexual capacity, or the ability to please a partner than is the size of a man's feet. Although some men worry that penis size is essential to being a good lover, the female genital organ most important to sexual arousal and orgasm is the clitoris, not the vagina, and it is more easily stimulated by touching with a hand than by thrusting with a penis.

As for intercourse, there is no scientific research suggesting that women generally prefer large penises, but there is research showing that most women generally do not care about their sexual partner's penis size. A vagina can feel stimulation in the 2 inches or so nearest the vaginal opening, so physiologically a penis that reaches this area is adequate for vaginal stimulation.

Some of these concerns may derive from the way men visually compare their own penises to those of other men. A man should realize that his own penis may look smaller than those of other men because of the viewing angle. Looking down at one's penis, it appears shorter than when viewed from the side or front, the way one might see the genitals of other men in locker rooms or public toilets.

During puberty there is an additional problem with such observations because not all boys' genitals begin to neither grow at the same age nor do they grown at the same rate. However, by adulthood, the boys who developed later or more slowly catch up. Unfortunately, many young men have made unfavorable comparisons before they've reached full growth and the thought that they're "small" says in their heads even after they've reached a fully mature average size. Because it is also during adolescence that we begin to interact with others and practice the social skills we need to function healthily in adult relationships, men should seek counseling help when they first begin to feel inadequate, rather than postponing it.

Even in early childhood, a young boy is likely to compare his penis to his father's and begin worrying about smallness. Parents can take steps to stop these worries before they even start.

If an adult is concerned and finds upon measuring his penis 2 inches or less when erect, he should have an evaluation by a urologist to see if there is a correctable problem involved.

But any man who feels self-conscious, humiliated, frustrated, depressed, embarrassed, anguished, angry, or suicidal because he thinks his penis is too short—whatever the size actually is—should talk with a counselor, psychologist, or psychiatrist. Although there is no product to increase the size of the penis, therapy can indeed boost a man's self-esteem and help him understand that his body is just fine the way it is.

Penile Injury

Q. I have read that one shouldn't use vacuum devices advertised to enlarge the penis, because they can damage erectile tissue.

If such damage has already occurred to penile tissue, can it be surgically repaired, or is the damage irreversible? This affects me directly. What action should be taken? This is very frustrating. Your answer will help put an end to my mental and physical suffering.

Ans. Repair depends on exactly what is wrong with the penis. You will have to consult a specialist in male sexual functioning who is skilled in assessing male genital problems resulting from trauma or injury to the penis. The specialist, usually a urologist, can evaluate your condition and discuss treatment options. It is very important that you explain precisely what happened. If you still have the device, take it with you so the physician can better understand all the factors involved. Most urologists have heard about these vacuum pumps and treated injury caused by them; so don't feel too embarrassed to seek help.

Largest Penis

Q. My question may seem very strange and odd, but I am curious about this. Concerning the size of penises: What is the largest size penis on record?

Ans. The blue whale reportedly has the largest penis, approximately 10 feet long. The longest erect human penis on record is 14 inches, documented early in the twentieth century by Dr. Robert L. Dickinson, a physician interested in sex research.

Large Penis and Young Girls

Q. I am a 20-year-old man who is having trouble having sex with young ladies because I have an overly large penis. It seems to hurt them too much. Have you ever heard of this problem? What can be done?

Ans. Are you sure the size of your penis is the problem here? Before assuming you're too large, consider some other possibilities. Maybe your partners weren't fully aroused before you attempted penetration. When a woman is sexually excited her vagina becomes lubricated and expands, making intercourse more comfortable, so that insertion and thrusting are not painful. For most women adequate foreplay is an essential part of lovemaking.

In addition to not penetrating until your partner is fully sexually aroused, you might want to try positions in which the woman can control the depth of penetration and movements. This means having your partner on top or being side-by-side. Whatever position you choose, ask whether your partner is ready to begin intercourse and let her control insertion so she can use an angle that's comfortable for her. If she feels discomfort or pain, stop deep or hard thrusting. Many women find shallow and gentle thrusting more pleasurable. If trying different techniques doesn't work, consult a sex counselor, who can offer suggestions that are specific to you and your partner.

Unequal Breasts

Q. I am 42 and have asymmetrical breasts (my left breast is larger than my right breast). It has been this way for most of my life since my breasts developed, but the older I get the worse it becomes. It's now to the point that it is difficult to find clothing that doesn't make me look lopsided. Do I have any medical recourse other than breast augmentation to correct the unevenness or is this a stump doctors know nothing about?

Ans. You have four options: augmentation mammoplasty surgery to increase the size of the smaller breast; reduction mammoplasty to reduce the size of the larger breast; camouflage the size difference with clothing and by padding one bra cup; or have counseling to learn to accept your body as it is. If you elect surgery, find a good, qualified, experienced cosmetic or plastic surgeon.

Most women's breasts are at least somewhat uneven, and many women imagine that differences between their breasts in size or shape are much more noticeable than they really are. A conscientious physician will discourage surgery if it is not necessary for the improvement of your appearance.

Enlarged Male Breasts

Q. I'm a 25 years man. I weigh 190 pounds and am 6 feet tall. Basically, I'm built quite well except I have large breasts. It's most embarrassing when I wear tight shirts. For many years I've hoped I could do something about this problem. But I've never done anything. Please send any information that would be helpful.

PS: I'm trying to tell you that I'd like to have my breasts made smaller, some way, so that I could wear tight shirts without embarrassment. Please help.

Ans. Enlargement of the male breast (gynecomastia) is not unusual and can have many causes, each with appropriate treatments. Make an appointment with an endocrinologist to evaluate your condition.

Researchers estimate that between 30 percent and 40 percent of all men over age seventeen have breast enlargement great enough to warrant the medical label of gynecomastia.

It is important to have a physical examination to rule out major problems such as tumors of the adrenal glands and the testicles, which can alter hormone levels. Some diseases such as cirrhosis of the liver (from excess alcohol consumption) and kidney failure, as well as malnutrition, can cause breast enlargement in men, as can a number of drugs (including reserpine, digitalis, and spironolactone).

When a disease is found and treated or a suspected drug is changed, the condition lessens for some men, but not for all. If an endocrinologist finds that you are generally healthy and you truly want to have your breasts reduced, then ask to be referred to a plastic or cosmetic surgeon who specializes in breast reduction. The results can be quite natural looking with nipple sensitivity retained and minimal scarring.

Any man who notices sudden breast enlargement should consult a physician promptly. While simple gynecomastia may be involved, in other cases breast tumors can be the cause. Since men, like women, can develop breast cancer, every man should regularly examine his breasts for lump or changes.

A final related point. Many newborn male babies have breast enlargement for a few weeks (probably because of exposure to the mother's estrogen) and about 60 percent to 70 percent of boys experience temporary breast growth during puberty due to fluctuations in the levels of androgens and estrogen.

Hairless Body

Q. I am male, 37 years old. But I look like I am 25-26 years of age. My problem is that I have no body hair. Is there a drug, which causes hair to grow? I am in excellent health. Should I consult a doctor?

Ans. If you want to have a hairier body because you assume women find it sexually attractive, you may be mistaken. Research has shown that most women rank hairiness low when rating physical components of male sexual attractiveness. I know of no effective drug approved to make body hair grow.

Hairy Nipples

Q. I am female, 34 years old. I want to know if the hair surrounding the nipples of my breasts is normal or unusual. When I nursed my first baby, the hospital nurse advised that I clip the hair so as not to annoy the baby. (I did not.) Does this hair, if not typical of most females, indicate a greater-than-normal amount of testosterone in my chemical make-up?

Ans. Many women have hair on their breasts. The amount of hair and its distribution on the body is controlled by several factors, the main one being heredity: Some people simply are hairier than other people, and darker hair shows up more than lighter hair.

Blood tests could determine if your hormone levels are within the normal range for women of your age.

Hair on the female chest area, however, is rarely associated with higher-than-normal levels of androgens ("male" hormones).

Plucking Nipple Hair

Q. Is it harmful to pluck hair from around the nipples?

Ans. No, but it can be painful and it's not a permanent solution. Hair will grow back after plucking. Nearly everyone has at least a few hairs around his or her nipples.

Role of Pubic Hair

Q. I am 18. I have very thick pubic hair, which my boyfriend wants me to shave. I hate the idea. I think of it as protection and fear I will feel funny and naked without it. What's the role of pubic hair? If I shave it, will it grow back again?

Ans. Pubic hair doesn't have a known biological function at this point in human history. But one theory holds that before people covered their bodies with clothing, pubic hair served to distribute pheromones (chemicals that carry specific messages to other members of the same species). These messages may have signaled, for instance, that a female was in her fertile stage. Growing a new crop of pubic hair after shaving can be very uncomfortable. It takes quite a while to get beyond the stubble stage, which can be itchy for you and irritating for your partner. But the best reason of all for not shaving it off is that you say you hate the idea. If you don't want to shave your pubic hair, don't. Your boyfriend should understand and respect your desire to leave your body the way it is.

Falling of Head Hair

Q. I am a 29-year-old male who's had a very active sex life since a teenager. For the last 2-½ years, I've noticed my head hair is thinning. Could the amount of sexual activity have anything to do with this?

Ans. It is highly unlikely that sexual activity would cause a man to lose his head hair, and there is also no research to either support or reject the widespread notion that bald men are "sexier."

Sudden hair loss can be a sign of a condition called alopecia areata (a scalp condition when hair falls out leaving bald patches), which requires diagnosis and treatment by a physician. Also, some disease accompanied by high fevers can cause hair loss, but in these cases the hair nearly always grows back. Other types of reversible hair loss include damage from hair products such as permanents or bleaches or by such drugs or medical treatments as cortisone, X-rays, or chemotherapy.

The vast majority of balding men have simply inherited the tendency to develop male-pattern baldness. About 12 percent of all men exhibit this type of gradual hair loss by age twenty-five, and nearly half of all men have significant hair loss by age forty-five.

Despite the many ads that promise growth of new hair, no drugs, lotions, vitamins, or other "miracle cures" have been shown to effectively reverse this type of hair loss in most men. One drug- minoxydil- helps some men. Before you consider using it, talk with your physician and make sure you understand the possible side effects, that it takes several months for this medication to begin to show results, and that if you stop using the medication any new hair will fall out.

There are also ways to camouflage a receding hairline or a bald spot, among them hairpieces, hair weaving, and hair plug transplants. When hair loss is viewed as a traumatic experience or has a negative effect on a man's ability to cope with life, counseling may be needed.

Masturbation

Q. I have a personal question to ask you. Is masturbation harmful to our health?

Ans. No, masturbation doesn't appear to be harmful to either physical or mental health.

Among the thousands of people interviewed by Kinsey during the 1940s and 1950s, 94 percent of males and 40 percent of females reported having masturbated to orgasm. More recent studies report that about the same percentage of males masturbate but that the percentage of females has increased to around 70 percent (or more, depending on the study).

Though masturbation is considered harmless. But still, it is also true, if done excessively it leads to premature ejaculation and ultimately ends up importancy.

Virginity

Q. I've been married for five years. On our wedding night, I discovered my wife was not a virgin. When I asked her about it, she said it was because she had been active in gymnastics in school, but she couldn't recall any specific accident when her hymen had been broken.

She assures me I'm the only man she has ever had intercourse with.

I love her and think she's a truthful person, but lately this question has been eating away at me. I'm depressed.

I've always assumed that penetration was required to rupture a hymen. Is it possible this could have happened without penetration?

Ans. Absolutely. The first act of intercourse for many women does not involve pain, bleeding, or any of the dramatic signs frequently thought to be associated with first intercourse. This is because the hymen has usually eroded. This natural process doesn't require penetration of any sort.

Even gynecologists doing pelvic examinations cannot usually tell if a woman is a virgin or not. And this can be true even when a hymen is found, since in some cases the tissue is so elastic it simply stretches during intercourse but does not tear. If a skilled physician who closely examines many women each day cannot usually establish virginity, it should come as no surprise that an untrained person cannot.

If you are truly depressed about this you should talk to a sex therapist. It's important to be able to trust your spouse, since many aspects of marriage must be based on trust.

Popular Positions

Q. What are the most popular positions for intercourse?

Ans. The most commonly used position in Western cultures is the so-called missionary position. There are many vaguely similar accounts about the origin of this term. One such story tells of a group of Pacific islanders who observed this sexual practice among Western missionaries and gave it that name, since it differed from their own usual position of having the woman on the top.

The woman-on-top position, with partners face-to-face and the woman either sitting up or lying down, is another common position for penile-vaginal intercourse. Others include face-to-face while lying side by side; and rear-entry positions, in which the man faces the woman's back while kneeling, sitting, standing, or lying down.

As with many other sexual activities, the choice of favourite intercourse position varies widely among individuals, couples, and even cultures. For example, the missionary position is among the most frequently used by couples in the United States, Japan, and some traditional groups in South America. Woman-on-top positions are more common than other positions among specific cultural groups in some of the South Pacific islands and sitting positions more common in tribal Australia. Various types of rear-entry positions are favored by couples of many groups, for example, the Marquesans in the Pacific.

Swallowing Semen

Q. I wonder if during oral sex, is it dangerous to swallow so many sperm at one time?

Ans. There is no evidence that swallowing semen (the fluid ejaculated by men at orgasm, which includes the sperm) is harmful to your health—unless the semen comes from someone who carries a disease that can be sexually transmitted. Diseases that can be transmitted by semen include gonorrhea, chlamydia, hepatitis B, and possibly the AIDS virus. Moreover, just having oral contact with the genitals (without swallowing semen) can transmit herpes, syphilis, and human papillomavirus. If these organisms are present

You should follow safer sex guidelines with partners unless you are certain they do not have an active stage of these diseases.

Lack of Sexual Desire (in Females)

Q. I'm a 40-year-old woman who for two years now has lost my sexual desire. My husband and I never had this problem for six years; in fact we had sex every chance we could. I just can't figure it out; I love my husband. Now he is lucky to make love to me once a month.

It seems I'm always tired. I've been to doctors, but they don't know what my problem is and I found it embarrassing to talk about. I know deep down my husband can't be happy with this new in me and he'll go to someone else.

Ans. Because you mention being tired, you should make an appointment with a sex dysfunction clinic that has physicians on staff or a specialist in gynecology for a complete checkup to rule out any underlying diseases or hormonal problems. When you call to make the appointment, tell the receptionist you've experienced a reduction in your previous level of sexual desire. Take along a list of all drugs you are taking, including vitamins, birth control pills, and nonprescription drugs such as tobacco and alcohol. Ask the doctor to review the list for possible sex-related side effects.

The most common health related causes of low sexual desire are depression, severe stress, side effects of drugs such as alcohol or high blood pressure medication, illnesses such as kidney disease, and changes in hormonal levels, especially testosterone. Any disruption of normal brain or nervous system activity can impair the physical mechanisms necessary for experiencing desire.

If no physical cause is found, you will then need an evaluation by a trained and experienced sex therapist or counsellor. Your husband will probably be asked to attend at least the first, appointment with you.

Lack of Sexual Desire (in Males)

Q. I'm 62, physically active, and in good health. However, my appetite for sex has diminished from once a week to once every two weeks. I can still perform once a week, but the appetite is missing. And, like with a good meal, the appetite is an important ingredient. This drop in frequency doesn't seem to matter to my wife. What kind of doctor should I see?

Ans. Any number of factors can affect sexual desire, including psychological causes (depression or stress), physical causes (a change in hormone levels, the side effect of a medication, or alcohol consumption), or a combination of these.

A substantial number of physically healthy men engage in sexual activity once every two weeks or even less frequently. According to one survey of more than 4000, age 50 or older, 75 percent of married men had sex once a week or less. However, some researchers suspect that the cultural expectation that older people should "slow down" may be as much of a factor as loss of actual desire or ability. Even though having sex every two weeks is neither unhealthy nor abnormal, if you're bothered by a decrease in sexual desire, it's time to seek expert help.

You say this change doesn't "seem" to matter to your wife. This suggests you haven't discussed it thoroughly with her. You may be surprised when you do. Communication is essential to a good sex life and a happy long-term marriage. Ask her to go along to your appointment and talk about each other's desires. By doing this your sex life may be improved even beyond its earlier level.

Alcohol and Sex

Q. I've read that alcohol can cause impotence, but I don't think that's true. I have better sex after I've had a few drinks. Why don't doctors just tell people with sex problems to drink?

Ans. Alcohol is a depressant drug and chemically acts to slow down, reduce, or stop the physical processes necessary for sexual arousal and orgasm. In men, alcohol can inhibit arousal, reduce erectile capacity, and slow or eliminate ejaculation and orgasm. In women, arousal, vaginal blood volume, and orgasm are all reduced with increased levels of alcohol.

Long-term alcohol use can lead to significant physical changes that can affect sexuality, some of which may be irreversible even if a person were to stop drinking. For example, alcohol consumption temporarily lowers testosterone levels and sperm counts in men. For men who drink regularly or on a prolonged basis, permanent sterility and testicular atrophy (shrinking) may result. Moreover, not only is testosterone lowered, but also estrogen (a "female" hormone) is increased, which can lead to irreversible breast enlargement (gynecomastia).

The amount that is harmful differs from one man or woman to the next, but similar effects on women who drink heavily have been noted, including atrophy of the ovaries, menstrual irregularities, and infertility.

Depressant drugs such as alcohol also have psychological effects. For some people this includes reducing sexual inhibitions, which may help a few individuals who feel shy or guilty to more freely express or experience their sexual desire and arousal. Others may use alcohol to excuse behavior that would be unacceptable to them when sober.

Physical and psychological reactions to alcohol vary widely from person to person. For example, 45 percent of the male respondents to a survey said that alcohol enhanced their sexual pleasure, but 42 percent reported that it decreased enjoyment.

Masters and Johnson describe a typical situation in which a man experienced an episode of high alcohol intoxication that resulted in erectile failure. The failure caused the man to become anxious about his sexual performance, which led to the use of more alcohol to lessen the anxiety, which led to further erection failures.

We also know alcohol can have a devastating effect on the fetus of a pregnant woman. For these and other reasons, anyone with sexual difficulties should consult a physician, therapist, or clinic rather than turning to beer, wine, or other liquors.

Lack of Testosterone

Q. I heard that a lack of testosterone hormone could keep a man away from performing. Can I get this hormone from changing my diet or do I need some pills to take?

Ans. Do you suspect your hormone level is too low? The only way to know whether this is the case is to have blood tests taken. If a blood test shows that you are deficient in testosterone, then taking supplemental testosterone might have some effect. But researchers have found that the effect is to increase sexual thoughts or fantasies rather than to increase erectile ability. Moreover, the physician would probably recommend injections, because testosterone in pill form is not as effective.

However, if your hormone level is normal, taking testosterone in any form is not likely to help and may actually do serious harm. One risk is that any undetected cancer in the prostate might be stimulated to grow.

I know of no dietary source of testosterone. Both pills and injections require prescription by a physician because these are powerful drugs with potentially serious mental and physical side effects that require careful monitoring while you use them.

Erection Problem

Q. I've always enjoyed sex with my wife, having fathered six children. Recently I've had trouble attaining and maintaining an erection it long enough to reach satisfaction. My wife understands my difficulty, but this is really bothering me when I can't follow up lovemaking with total satisfaction. My doctor tells me this is a "psychological problem" and that I have to work through it myself. But I don't seem to be making any progress.

Ans. For years, researchers felt that most erection problems were caused by purely psychological factors. But more recent studies have revealed that erectile difficulties can have many physical causes as well.

In one study 34 percent men were admitted having erectile difficulties. Of those who chose to be evaluated for this problem, the erection problems of only 14 percent were attributed to purely psychological causes. Twenty-eight percent were diagnosed as having various hormonal imbalances and 25 percent had erection problems caused by medications; other causes included diabetes, 9 percent; neurological (brain and nerves), 7 percent; urological (kidney, bladder, urethra), 6 percent; various other problems (such as the after effects of surgery) 4 percent. In only 7 percent of the cases was no specific cause found.

Therefore impotence is due to various causes and one rarely can work these problems out for himself you need to make an appointment at a clinic that specializes in diagnosis and treatment of sexual dysfunctions.

Quick Ejaculation and Circumcision

Q. I ejaculate very quickly, in less than a minute. Is it because I'm uncircumcised?

Ans. Uncircumcised men who ejaculate sooner than they would like often blaming the problem on having a foreskin, while many circumcised men who ejaculate too soon blame it on *not* having a foreskin. Neither assessment is valid, since each man's reactions to stimulation are not solely dependent on the presence or absence of a foreskin. Researchers have not found significant differences in sexual responses between these two groups of men.

Testosterone and Older People

Q. Is testosterone-replacement therapy something a man should consider, as he grows older?

Ans. Not as a matter of course. Testosterone, a hormone produced in higher amounts by men than by women, has been shown to decline with age for some men. But current medical thinking is that unless a man's testosterone levels is tested and found to be exceptionally low, there's no benefit in adding more and there many be negative mental and physical health-related side effects.

Research on men who took testosterone reported that there was some increase in the amount of sexual thoughts and fantasies, but there was no increase in erectile ability.

If you suspect a hormonal imbalance, ask your physician or an endocrinologist for a complete physical examination, including a screening for levels of testosterone and prolactin (a pituitary hormone). If you do need to take testosterone, make sure you follow the recommended schedule for prostate examinations. Changes in the prostate can be one side effect of taking testosterone.

Unequal Breasts

Q. I have a very serious problem I hope you can help me with. As I first developed breasts everything was "normal," but as they got bigger one breast became larger than the other.

I've been living with this problem for three years now. I've been doing breast exercises on just the smaller one but it doesn't seem to be getting any bigger. I'm too embarrassed to ask anybody about this in person.

Ans. Medical professionals have been saying for years that no woman has equal breasts; one is always slightly larger than the other. Some researchers now estimate that more than half of all women have visible size differences between their two breasts, and nearly one-fourth have one breast that is 20 percent larger than the other.

Exercise will not increase the amount of breast tissue in the smaller breast, although it could increase the underlying chest muscles so that the breast might appear a little larger. The best option is to overcome your embarrassment; it may help to remind yourself that millions of women have breasts like yours.

Fertility and age

Q. Are younger men more fertile than older men?

Ans. Men begin to produce sperm during puberty and, if healthy, continue to produce sperm until they die. Theoretically, a man can impregnate a woman at any age after he reaches puberty. In general, the number of sperm in each ejaculation is thought to be highest between ages 21 and 30.

However, many factors can temporarily reduce an individual male's sperm count. These include the length of time since the previous ejaculation, stress, fever, the temperature of the testicles, and infections of the reproductive organs.

The Cause of Single Baby in Humans

Q. Why do humans usually have only one baby at a time while dogs and cats have lots of babies at once?

Ans. Animals like dogs and cats have multiple births because they release several eggs in one reproductive cycle. Human females, on the other hand, usually release only one egg during each cycle.

Sperm Count Procedure

Q. My wife and I have been unable to conceive for over a year. After several examinations and tests

on her, our doctor has suggested a sperm count for me. What sort of procedure should I expect?

Ans. You will probably be told to have intercourse or masturbation for forty-eight to seventy-two hours before the test. You will then collect the semen sample by masturbating and ejaculating into a sterile glass container. The physician will provide a private area for you to collect your sample in the office.

Most fertility specialists recommend the masturbation method to collect sperm. Trying to withdraw during intercourse in time to ejaculate into the container is not though to be a good way to collect the semen since the first few drops, which contain the highest number of sperm, are often lost.

Collecting the semen by ejaculating into a condom is also not recommended, because many condoms contain a spermicidal, a lubricant, or ingredients for preservation of the latex, all of which can immobilize sperm or interfere with the test results. However, if a man's religion forbids masturbation, fertility clinics can provide a special type of condom made especially for this purpose.

The laboratory report on a basic analysis will contain several different types of information, including the volume of the semen, the number of viable (live) sperm, the consistency of the semen, the shape and health of the sperm, their ability to swim, and the presence of white blood cells that signify an infection someplace in the male reproductive tract.

A single semen evaluation, however, is not usually an adequate evaluation of male fertility, since many factors can temporarily increase or decrease the number of sperm. A high fever, for example, can reduce the number of healthy sperm in an ejaculation many weeks after the fever has occurred. So don't be surprised if the specialist asks for a second sample to be done a week or so later.

Vacuum devices and Penile Injury

Q. I have read that one shouldn't use vacuum devices advertised to enlarge the penis, because they can damage erectile tissue.

If such damage has already occurred to penile tissue, can it be surgically repaired, or is the damage irreversible? This affects me directly. What action should be taken? This is very frustrating. Your answer will help put an end to my mental and physical suffering.

Ans. Repair depends on exactly what is wrong with the penis. You will have to consult a specialist in male sexual functioning who is skilled in assessing male genital problems resulting from trauma or injury to the penis. The specialist, usually a urologist, can evaluate your condition and discuss treatment options. It is very important that you explain precisely what happened. If you still have the device, take it with you so the physician can better understand all the factors involved. Most urologists have heard about these vacuum pumps and treated injury caused by them; so don't feel too embarrassed to seek help.

Pregnancy and Menstruation

Q. I've heard that even if a woman is pregnant she can still have her menstrual flow. Is this true?

Ans. No, a pregnant woman does not continue to have her "true" menstrual flow. About 30 percent of women do have bleeding at some point during a pregnancy, but that bleeding is not menstruation. Even when bleeding occurs on exactly those days a woman would have expected to have her menstrual flow if she were not pregnant (which does happen to some women), it is considered to be different from menstruation. The amount of blood is usually less than the usual menstrual flow and lighter in color (pinkish rather than dark red).

One of the most common causes of bleeding in the early weeks of pregnancy results from implantation of the embryo in the lining of the uterus (a normal process). In some women, however, bleeding can be a sign that the placenta is not producing enough progesterone or that there's an irritation or infection of the cervix or vagina. Sometimes, strenuous activity or a fall can jar the uterus enough to cause bleeding from the placenta. Or bleeding can be the first signal of a serious medical emergency—for example, an ectopic pregnancy (when the embryo implants and begins to grow in a Fallopian tube or location other than the uterus).

For these reasons, all bleeding during pregnancy must be reported to your physician immediately. If the bleeding is accompanied by pain or cramping and you cannot reach your physician, go to a hospital emergency room.

Making Love during Pregnancy

Q. Does making love during pregnancy hurt the baby or the mother?

Ans. There is no scientific evidence that sexual intercourse at any stage of pregnancy harms the vast majority of mothers or babies. Those couples whose pregnancy ended in miscarriage should understand that it is extremely unlikely that sexual activity was a direct cause of the loss.

There are, however, a few exceptions to this general rule. For example, if the woman has vaginal bleeding, pain, or leakage of amniotic fluid, sexual intercourse should be discontinued until a physician advises otherwise. Women who have a history of premature labor and delivery or miscarriages, or whose cervix has already dilated, may be cautioned against having intercourse or told to use a condom. The uterine contractions associated with an orgasm may induce labor, which can be a problem if the fetus is not fully developed. On the other hand, orgasm is one nonchemical way to initiate the uterine contractions needed for delivery at the end of the full gestation period.

Moreover the prostaglandins in semen may induce uterine contractions in some women—another reason for using a condom.

Studies have compared babies born to women who continued sexual intercourse throughout pregnancy with those of women who stopped having intercourse at some point in the pregnancy. Research also has compared babies born to mother who reported having orgasms, with babies whose mothers didn't have orgasms. In both studies, researchers found no significant differences among these babies on any measures of infant health.

However, for complete safety, there are two sexual practices that women must avoid during pregnancy: (1) Forcefully blowing air into the vagina (which should never be done) can cause an embolism (an air bubble), which can lead to death of the mother and fetus, and (2) having sex with someone who carries a sexually transmitted disease, which can lead to fetal defects, disease, and in some case death, depending on which STD organism is involved.

Not all pregnant women are interested in having sex, and some are interested in sex during some points of the pregnancy but not at others. Research by Master and Johnson on pregnant women revealed a decreased desire for sex in the first trimester (months one to three), a rise in sexual interest in the second trimester (months four to six), and a gradual decline in the third trimester (month seven to birth). Other researchers report different patterns of sexual activity or interest in sex. Many books on pregnancy simply state that sexual desire and activity during pregnancy varies widely from one woman to the next.

Tight Foreskin

Q. When I have a full erection, my foreskin retracts as it should, but the sensation isn't very pleasing. It feels very tight. I also have trouble retracting it myself when I want to wash. Is circumcision the only solution to my problem?

Ans. The alternative to complete circumcision is a very minor slit in the foreskin; it's called a "dorsal slit." That can be done in the doctor's office, in a matter of minutes, under a little local anesthetic.

The anesthetic is injected at the top of the foreskin. To visualize that, picture 12 o'clock on a dial. Two small mosquito forceps are then put on the foreskin and a small cut—one quarter to three eights on an inch long-made. The clamps are left on for five or six minutes so that there will be no bleeding, and then removed.

You could not have intercourse for several days-five or six at least-until the slits are healed enough so that there would be no danger of bleeding.

The operation would enlarge the opening of the foreskin so that it would then retract without any sense of tightness whatever.

The only thing for you to do is to consult a urologist. Be sure you get one who is willing to do a dorsal slit, and who will not insist that the only thing to do is to have a complete circumcision. The latter is totally unnecessary if you do not want it.

Oral Sex Normal?

Q. My husband and I enjoy a happy sex life. Some time back, when he was a little intoxicated, he performed oral sex upon me. I enjoyed it very much, but he has avoided doing it again. He says he wants to please me, but is afraid that such acts are not normal, and that they may be harmful, too. Does oral sex harm the body in any way?

Ans. Oral contacts with both the male and female genitals are perfectly normal and harmless. If they give either or both of you greater satisfaction and pleasurable stimulation, there is no reason why you should not continue mouth-genital contact.

Forever Sterile?

Q. I am over 21. I am about to marry a man who had a vasectomy during his first marriage. Will this make him sterile forever? I have heard that the operation can be undone. Is this true?

Ans. It is true that when a man has had a vasectomy a surgeon can try to restore his fertility by another operation. The rate of success is not high.

If his fertility is restored, you should try to have a child as soon as possible. The difficulty is that scar tissue can form slowly and contract, so that even if the second operation were successful his sperm ducts might become blocked after a few months.

If the operation fails, you might want to consider either artificial insemination or adoption.

Penis Lubrication

Q. When I am aroused by my fiancée, the head of my penis becomes very wet. I suppose that this lubrication is normal, but what I want to know is whether there are sperm in this fluid that could make a girl pregnant. Is it safe to insert my penis into her vagina in foreplay, before I put on a condom?

Ans. When a man is aroused sexually, there is usually some lubrication that comes from the glands along the urethra. However, there may also be a slight spillover of sperm from the seminal vesicles, so that a t times this pre-coital fluid will contain sperm.

It is always risky to insert the penis into the vagina if adequate contraceptive measures have not been taken. Girls have become pregnant from pre-coital fluid, even though the man was careful enough to put on a condom before starting actual intercourse. It is a strange thing, but while some men are infertile because of a low sperm count, others have unintentionally become fathers due to the presence of just a few sperm in their lubricating fluid.

Stretch Marks

Q. I have veins on my stomach. They come from having a baby, and I was told that they would go away after six months. But my baby is a year old now and the veins are still there. How can I get rid of them?

Ans. I wonder if you are not describing little stripes, bands, or lines rather than veins. These are a slightly different color than the skin around them, and may be slightly depressed. They are called stria. If that is what you are referring to, there is no way to get rid of them. It is just something you will have to accept.

Erection After Coitus

Q. I am 23. Sometimes when I have intercourse my penis stays erect after I ejaculate, and I can continue intercourse for several minutes longer. At other times, I lose my erection almost immediately after orgasm. Is there anything wrong with me? I have never heard of a man staying erect for a while after ejaculation.

Ans. It is not unusual for a young man's erection to continue for a short time after ejaculation. Loss of erection right after orgasm is the more general experience, however.

If you have intercourse frequently, you might lose your erection right after orgasm. It could be a matter of how much sexual tension has been built up, and how fully the tension has been discharged by orgasm. The way you feel emotionally at any particular time that you have intercourse would play a part in this, too.

Whether your penis stays erect for a time after ejaculation, or becomes limp right away, is not important. You have nothing to worry about so long as intercourse is satisfactory to you and your partner.

Menopause Symptoms

Q. I am 39, married, and have three children. I have heard that some women go through the menopause between the ages of 40 and 50. Can you tell me what the symptoms are?

I get pains in my stomach and left side, and sweat once in a while. Are these menopause symptoms?

Ans. Some women enter menopause before 40. The principal symptoms are a certain amount of emotional upset without any particular cause, and a decrease in the amount of menstrual flow. Hot flashes are very common. The individual gets red in the face and perspires a great deal, then feels quite cool a few minutes later.

I do not believe that either the pain in your stomach or your left side is necessarily connected with menopause. I would urge you to consult your doctor. Female sex hormone, estrogen, can help a woman who is suffering from menopause symptoms. It should be taken only by prescription.

Regaining "Virginity"

Q. **I have heard that girls who have lost their virginity can have it restored by an operation. Is this true? What does the doctor do in such cases?**

Ans. Virginity cannot be restored. Once the penis has penetrated the vagina, the woman can no longer be considered a virgin.

What can be restored is a woman's hymen. The operation is very simple and can be done in a doctor's office. An anesthetic is injected at the torn edges of the hymen. They are snipped clean so that there is a fresh, slightly bleeding surface. This is then sewn together. After healing has taken place, the woman once again has an intact hymen.

Breast-Enlargement Danger

Q. I am 20 and married. I would like to have larger breasts. I've read that silicone shots will do this. Can you tell me if that is true? Is the operation complicated? Is it expensive?

Ans. Silicone injections to make women's breasts larger were very fashionable some years ago, but this method has been discarded as unsafe. The results turned out to be disastrous in many cases, and for that reason the method is illegal in some countries.

If you wish to have your breasts enlarged, the only safe way is to have an operation. It is done by a plastic surgeon, who places a plastic sac containing silicone jell beneath the breasts. You can have whatever size breasts you wish, and the doctor will advise you as to what is best in your case.

The operation is moderately expensive and you will need to spend four or five days in the hospital. In some patients who have a deficiency of female hormone, estrogen treatment can be moderately successful in increasing bust size.

Genital Odor

Q. I am 21 and married. I wash my genitals carefully every day, and use my fingers to make sure that all the vaginal creases and folds are clean. But my husband says that my vagina has an odor that makes it almost impossible for him to make love to me. What can be done about this?

Ans. The thing for you to do is consult a gynecologist to see what causes the unpleasant odor from your vagina. A yeast or trichomonas infection could be the cause. You might also have a cervical erosion of course these conditions can be cured, but a careful examination is needed to discover what is producing the odor.

Wife Lacks Passion

Q. **I am 65 and my wife is 60. My wife is very accommodating. She has climaxes occasionally but is not as passionate as I would like her to be. She does not seem to have much sexual desire. Do you think that vitamins, special foods, hormones, or a vibrator would help?**

Ans. Since your wife seems willing to see to it that you are taken care of sexually, I think you have a great deal to be thankful for.

She could possibly obtain more pleasure herself if she realizes that not only does the mind affect the body but also the body affects the mind.

The more active a part she takes in sexual activity, the more she is likely to get out of it herself. In turn, your satisfaction and pleasure will be increased.

It might help your wife if she let her imagination run riot, and do everything and anything that might occur to her. It is not too late for you both to experiment with anything that seems pleasing. A vibrator might be useful but not vitamins, special food or hormones.

Penetration Pain

Q. **My wife and I have tried several intercourse positions, but when I fully insert my penis she finds it painful. It feels to me as if I am pushing against something in her vagina.**

We went to a gynecologist, but he couldn't find anything wrong with her. He did say that she was built "small." We always engage in enough foreplay

so that our organs are thoroughly wet. What is my wife's problem?

Ans. If your wife's uterus is tipped backward and bound down—a retroverted uterus—then you might be hitting the bottom of it. That could be painful for her. If one of her ovaries has falledn down-a prolapsed ovary—then hitting that could hurt her. If, due to the retroverted uterus, your penis is striking above her cervix instead of below and behind it, then that would be painful for her.

If she kneels on the edge of the bed and lies forward, with her chest resting on the bed, this rear-entry position might be helpful. Everything would tend to fall upward in her abdominal cavity, and deep penetration might be possible without pain.

In face-to-face intercourse, if she brings her legs slightly together, and you put your legs outside hers, you could thrust as hard as you like without hurting her. This position prevents deep penetration.

I suggest that your wife see another gynecologist inasmuch as the gynecologist she first went to found nothing wrong. Obviously, a problem does exist.

Genital Infection

Q. About a month ago I acquired a very irritating itch in the areas of my rectum, inner and outer vaginal lips, and clitoris. I have a vaginal discharge that is sometimes white, sometimes clear. When I scratch those areas, a strong, and unpleasant odor results. The only relief I have been able to get is from a cream claimed to stop itching. But the relief is only temporary—the irritation returns after a few hours. What is it? How did I get it?

Ans. What you describe are certainly symptoms of a yeast, or monilia, infection of the vagina. What you should do is consult a gynecologist. If your trouble is monilia, it can go away by itself. If there is some other cause, a competent examination should uncover it.

Where a yeast infection comes from is something we cannot be sure about. It could be transmitted through intercourse.

If your husband is not circumcised and carries the yeast organism beneath his foreskin, then he could infect you. If his condition is not cleared up, he could reinfect you every time you have intercourse with him. For this reason, I suggest both of you consult your physician for an examination.

Sex Techniques

Q. During sex relations with my wife I always have to manipulate her clitoris until she reaches orgasm. My wife says that during relations my penis never touches her clitoris. As far as I can see, what we are doing amounts to masturbation; only I am doing it to her instead of she doing it to her self. Will this endanger her health and make her sterile?

Ans. It does not matter in the least how you bring your wife to reach orgasm. The important thing is that she enjoys relations and does reach orgasm. Anything that you can do in any way that helps her to reach orgasm is not only perfectly all right and permissible, but highly desirable. Neither masturbation nor this sort of stimulation can hurt her in any way.

Ovulation Pain

Q. Do pain and some discharge have anything to do with the releasing of an egg? Sometimes around the middle of my menstrual cycle I feel a little

pain and have a tiny discharge, but not nearly like the menstrual discharge.

Ans. It is not at all unusual for a woman to have just a little, almost a pricking or stinging pain, for a short time-and occasionally there will be a slight bloody discharge, enough so that it would be noticed on toilet paper once or twice. That is the signal of ovulation. That means that an egg has been discharged from a follicle in an ovary. This usually happens on the 10th to 13th day following the onset of menstruation.

Semen Odor

Q. **I am unmarried, 43, and have no sexual outlets. I have not masturbated for a number of years, but several times a month I have involuntary orgasms and emissions. These usually occur after I have been asleep for a few hours.**

My concern is with the semen. It is so strong smelling that it penetrates the whole room and even outside to the corridors and other rooms. Washing myself still doesn't entirely remove the odor.

This troubles me. It is unsanitary and I don't want people to think I masturbate. I like to be clean and not offend others. I know sex and semen are not dirty, and the right use of sex is beautiful, I suppose. I've never experienced a sex act, so I cannot tell, but I sense that only in marriage can it rise to true heights of beauty and spirituality.

For an unmarried man like myself, though, I would like to stop these emissions or at least neutralize the odor. Is there any way I can do this?

Ans. You are, of course, far too concerned about these emissions. They are an entirely harmless and normal release from sexual tensions. The odor is probably detectable only to you because of your deep concern and preoccupation.

Semen, of course, does have a definite odor but it should not be anything like as strong as you seem to indicate that yours is. If this is so, then there must be some cause for it. It is possible that you have a low grade prostatic infection which contributes to it. You can consult a urologist and have a through examination to see if he could come up with a possible explanation.

Small Penis

Q. I am 21 years old and have never had sexual relations. My penis and testes are smaller than normal and I have always thought that sexual intercourse would cause these organs to grow to normal size. However, I recently was told this is not true. Since I will soon be married I would like to know if I could expect to have a larger penis after intercourse. Mine is about 4 ½ inches when erect.

Ans. Sexual intercourse will not increase the size of the penis. The only thing that might possibly have changed that might have been to have some adequate.

Hormonal treatment during the growth years back in the teens. However, size is for the most part determined by heredity, and except for rarer cases of hormone deficiency, nothing could be done at any age. If you would like, you can get the opinion of an endocrinologist a doctor who specializes in glands and hormones. The loving attention, the kindness, consideration, and thoughtfulness that you can show your wife is far more important than the size of the penis. A penis that is 4 ½ " long will serve perfectly satisfactorily as a copulative organ.

Enlarged Breasts

Q. My breasts have become enlarged. I have not tried to decrease their size, but if I should desire to do so is there a drug to take for this purpose? What causes this increase in size?

Ans. There is no drug that would decrease the size of your breasts. It may be that you have gained some weight and that you simply have had an increase in the size of the fat pad of the breast. Generally, enlargement of a man's breasts is carefully checked out by a doctor because it may be due to disturbed liver function.

Hymen Absent

Q. I am girl of 18. Recently my finance persuaded me to elope with him without the knowledge of my parents. The tragedy was that I had no hymen. I never had sex relations with a man before and I swore to this to my husband, but he didn't believe me and we parted. Now he wants to be together again as a man and wife, but I fear he will always have some doubt. I am and always have been a descent girl. I will keep your answer as proof of my innocence.

Ans. It is not at all unusual for a girl to be born without a hymen. Some are born with only a very small hymen, or one that is so easily stretched that no bleeding or pain whatever occurs at first intercourse. Your husband should not doubt you at all solely on this basis.

Seminal Fluid

Q. Does the prostate gland produce and them store its fluid in the seminal vesicles so that all the fluid comes from the vesicles at ejaculation? Or do they both secrete fluid at ejaculation?

Ans. Both the prostate gland and the seminal vesicles secrete fluid. The prostate contributes its fluid at the moment of orgasm, and the seminal vesicles do also. It is this mixture of the two, which activates the sperm, which are at least in part stored in the seminal vesicles prior to ejaculation.

Retaining Semen

Q. I am trying to become pregnant. Assuming that ovulation time has been taken into consideration, will intercourse in a face-to-face position increase the possibility of becoming pregnant?

Ans. If your womb is in normal position, meaning that it tips forward over the bladder with the neck of the womb slanting somewhat toward your back, then lying on your back is the best position. The pool of semen after orgasm then collects in the lower portion of the vagina with the cervix (womb neck) in it so that sperm have the best possibility of making their way into the womb. It is helpful to lie on your back and not walk about for some time after intercourse in order to retain the ejaculate.

Smegma Secretion

Q. I have to get married very soon because my fiancée refuses to wait any longer. But I have a problem.

Around the glans of my penis a white substance is secreted that has a bad odor if it isn't washed every day. I am ashamed to get married and expose my wife in this bad smell. Do you think circumcision help?

Ans. Circumcision would help avoid the secretion, called smegma, which you mention. The easier thing to do is, of course, to carefully remove this by washing at least once a day to avoid the unpleasant odor.

Erections in Sleep

Q. My problem is that for the past 2 years I have been getting strong erections while I am sleeping. Sometimes they awaken me. Frequently, I feel exhausted and can't put myself completely into my work. Could this be because the sex erections drain my energy?

Ans. It is quite common to have erections during sleep, and although it is not really known why, they may be quite associated from sexual arousal. In investigating nocturnal emissions, the Kinsey group learned that men sometimes even ejaculate in their sleep while having dreams involving nonsexual activities. Sometimes, also, men even ejaculate in their sleep with no memory of dreaming or thinking anything. Their opinion, which goes with the view of most psychiatrists, is that people are unable to recall the dreams, which they were having. This may be case with your erections. It is also contended by some that the stimulations of a full bladder sexual nerves creates erection during sleep.

At any rate, these erections probably have nothing to do with your feelings of exhaustion-that is, unless you are losing sleep worrying about them. Fatigue could be due to any number of possible causes. The only thing for you to do is to see a doctor and have a thorough physical examination.

Sex Changes

Q. Is it easier for a male to become a female through surgery than for a female to become a male? How can a female be made to seem like a male?

Ans. It is very definitely easier for a male to be made to appear as a female through surgery than for a female to become a male. The penis and scrotum can be removed and an artificial vagina can be created between the base of the penis behind the pubic bone and in front of the rectum.

It is almost impossible to construct a penis because the mechanism which brings about an erection is a delicate thing. At least one attempt was made to fashion a copulatory organ by suing a piece of rib. This started out apparently to be successful, but then the whole thing sloughed off and it failed. Females can of course receive male hormone treatments from a Doctor, which can bring about a deeper voice and more masculine hair distribution and small penis. But there are great individual differences in response.

Waning Potency

Q. I am 75 years old and married to a young woman. I am partially impotent-that is, my penis does not reach full erection and I cannot satisfy the sexual cravings of my wife. I want to know if there is any device that can be attached to my sexual organ to help me perform coitus. Do you know of any effective treatment to restore potency? I am willing to pay any price.

Ans. Since you are 75 years of age, you are, of course, at an age where some men do become impotent. Occasionally, if a person is capable of even a slight erection, placing a rubber band snugly around the base of the penis may make it possible for him to maintain an erection sufficient to carry on sex relations. Of course it would be worth your while to consult a sexologist and see if the administration of male sex hormone might also prove of some help. It might not do the least bit of good, but on the other hand it might and so is worth trying.

Swollen Testicles

Q. My testicles are swollen and harder than normal due to masturbating too frequently or to an injury sustained while playing football. The right testicle has a distinct, though not sharp, pain. It has been swollen for the part 3 months. I am afraid this may lead to sterility or impotence. What could be wrong with me?

Ans. You should consult a physician preferably an urologist. It may be nothing more than a hydrocele, which is an accumulation of fluids around the testicle, or possibly even a varicocele, which is a swelling of the veins leading from the testicles. In either case it could be corrected by operation. It is not likely that masturbation would have caused any such trouble. If you were Injured by a sever blow in football, it might have contributed to the difficulty. But by all means do consult a physician, and on the basis of an adequate examination have a diagnosis, upon which some treatment might be based.

Inheriting Dwarfism

Q. What causes some people to become dwarfs? Is this defect hereditary? I intend to marry a young woman who is 5'5" tall and who has ten brothers who are perfectly normal, but also has an uncle-her mother's brother-who is a dwarf. If I married this girl, could my children be dwarfs?

Ans. A young woman who is 5'5" is a good average height for a young woman. Since all her brothers are quite normal and a dwarf is a brother of her mother, it may well be that something happened in this childhood to stunt his growth and it is not what is termed a congenital or inborn defect.

There would appear to be very little danger of having a child who would be a dwarf if you were to marry this girl. One cannot, of course, say that it could not happen because it might occur for some other reason rather than purely hereditary.

Peyronie's Disease

Q. During the past two years my penis has become more and more crooked when erect. It bends to the left beginning at about the middle of it and there is a hardened ridge along the top. My doctor says it is peyronie's disease.

Is it known what causes this condition? Can it be cured and is it considered serious? So far it does not seem to cause any discomfort.

Ans. The cause of Peyronie's disease is not definitely known. It is a degeneration of the spongy tissue of the penis. Until quite recently, it was thought that there was little that could be done for it. Now in the hands of a very competent urologist it is possible to do a great deal of good through operation. The fibrous portion is removed and the normal shape of the penis resorted. If the curvature of the penis is not too great so that intercourse is not interfered with, it is probably better to do nothing at all.

Life of Sperm

Q. Does sperm lose its potency after hitting the air? If it does not lose its ability to impregnate a woman the second it is exposed to air, how does it take?

Ans. The mere fact that semen was exposed to the air momentarily would not mean that the sperm would be killed or destroyed. So long as they are still in the fluid medium of the semen, they would be alive and probably capable of fertilization.

There are cases of pregnancy occurring where the vagina has not actually been entered by the penis, but ejaculation merely taken place at the vaginal entrance. In this way, even a girl who is still a virgin and whose hymen is still intact may become pregnant.

Virginity

Q. I am going to get married very shortly and I would like to know if my husband can tell for sure if I'm a virgin or not. If it doesn't hurt and bleed a lot, will he have every right to point the finger of shame and perhaps leave me?

Ans. There is no way that one can tell positively whether or not a girl has had sex relations. Frequently physicians themselves are unable to tell. At least 30 per cent of all young women when they marry have so elastic a hymen that first intercourse does not cause any pain or any bleeding.

It would seem to me that you are laying altogether too much stress on this. If a man is marrying a girl because he is in love with her, the important thing is that he loves the girl whether or not she might previously have had sexual intercourse.

Irregular Periods

Q. I am 34 years old. My periods used to be 28 days apart and they would last for seven days. But more than a year ago I was pregnant and had a miscarriage after three months. Afterwards, I had a dilation and curettage (scraping of the womb) done.

Ever since that miscarriage, my periods haven't been regular. They may come anywhere from nine to twenty days apart. I have cramps when the periods begin, but otherwise I feel fine. My doctor had me on hormone shots and thyroid pills, but they didn't help. Now my doctor has moved away. Do you think it's important for me to see another gynecologist? Could it be that I am having my change of life?

Ans. We can only advise you to, by all means, consult a competent gynecologist. If you are menstruating so irregularly and particularly with a frequency of from nine to twenty days, this should certainly be looked into. It is utterly impossible for us to give you any other advice.

Discharge from Penis

Q. When I have a bowel movement I have noticed that a white penile discharge occurs. What causes this?

Ans. The white discharge that appears at the head of the penis following movement is undoubtedly some secretion squeezed out of the seminal vesicles or the prostate by the fecal (bowel) matter passing over them.

Scrotal Cysts

Q. I have noticed for many years that the bag my testicles are in has a larger number of white lumps under the skin. Some are as large as a pencil eraser. What are they? Are they serious?

Ans. The large lumps in the skin of your scrotum are undoubtedly small sebaceous cysts. This is not serious, occasionally one of them may become infected and cause some trouble. You would be wise to consult an urologist regarding this and follow what treatment he suggests.

Rh Blood Factor

Q. I have Rh-positive blood. If I marry a man with Rh-negative blood will it affect our children we have? Please clear this up for me.

Ans. Where the husband is Rh negative and wife Rh positive there is never any danger to the child. It is only where the mother is Rh negative and the father is Rh positive that trouble may result. Even in this latter situation there is difficulty only in one out of every thirty couples that have that combination. So the danger, in any event is not very great. For those cases where there is difficulty, blood transfusions for the child are necessary.

Varicocele

Q. I have hernia and during the past few years I have noticed a swelling that periodically appears in the upper right side of my penis. When I touch the left side of my scrotum. I feel formations of something similar to tubes. My doctor advises an operation. Which I will have after I get married about seven months from now. What do you think is wrong with me?

Ans. From your description of the swelling beside the penis and in the scrotum, you must have what is called a varicocele. These are simply distended veins. They can be operated upon and removed without any too great difficulty.

It would probably be wiser to have it done before you are married rather afterwards. If your marriage were still seven months away you would have ample time to have this done.

Infertile Husband

Q. For six years I have been trying to become pregnant. The gynecologist I went to said I am in perfect physical condition. But my husband had his sperm examined and the test showed that his sperm is weak; that is, he doesn't produce enough sperm. Could I use some sort of injector to introduce my husband's sperm well inside my womb? Do you think it could be harmful?

Ans. One would have to have some definite information as to just what is the status of the sperm activity and the sperm count of your husband's semen before any adequate recommendation could be made. Why do you not consult your own gynecologist or your husband's urologist and get this specific information?

It is unwise to introduce semen directly into the womb. The only thing that can be done is to be sure that semen is introduced close to the womb mouth (cervix) or just barely within the cervical opening. If it is put up into the womb itself, it might set up a reaction that would be painful and defeat the purpose of such an injection.

Breast Growth

Q. I am 24 years old, married, with two children. I nursed my last child for eleven months. For the three years following her weaning, my breasts seems to grow larger and heavier every day. This is very disturbing and, to say the least, very uncomfortable. Is there an operation of some kind or even some medicine that can stop the growth or shrink the breasts?

Ans. A physician to make certain that there is no serious cause such as cysts or tumors should certainly look into the increase in breast size. First of all your gynecologist should certainly look for any cyst or tumor in your breasts. On the other hand, this may be serious.

But there may well be a harmless cause such as obesity. You did not give us any information as to how much weight you have gained since you weaned your last child. Have you gained a considerable amount? If you have then the increased size of your breasts is probably due merely to the increase in fat around glandular portion of the breasts. Also it is possible to have plastic surgery done over the breasts. There was a great vogue of this some twenty-give years ago. The results are apt to be disappointing in that the breasts sometimes become lumpy and lose their smooth, soft contour. Surgery would not be advisable unless it becomes very necessary.

Size Concern

Q. My question may sound stupid, but believe me it is very important. I am nineteen years old and married. I would like to know if there is any way to make a male's penis larger-any way at all. I am six feet tall. I weigh 70 Kg., built very well. When my penis is erect it is only five inches. It makes me feel like I am small when my wife and I are having sex relations. This is really hurting my personality and giving me an inferiority complex. Your answer will be appreciated. Thank you very much.

Ans. Since your penis is five inches long when erect, it is at the longer edge of average, which is considered between five and six inches. It is not at all unusual for a larger man to have a relatively small penis and a small man to have a very large penis. However, both you and your wife should be made to understand that size is of little importance in making a man a competent sex partner. The sexually sensitive areas of the female require very little or no penetration for stimulation.

Since you are only nineteen, there is a very faint possibility that if you take adequate hormonal treatment it might increase the size of your penis somewhat, although it is doubtful. The thing for you to do is to consult an endocrinologist and see what he might have to suggest. Penis size is determined by heredity, for the most part. Your wife certainly should stop making any remarks of a disparaging nature even though it might come in the form of 'kidding'. She should say or do nothing to call this to your attention and thereby hurt you. It might help to clear the air if you were to talk the whole matter over with her calmly and sensibly.

Coital Duration

Q. I have a very important question that I would like to get some advice on. When my wife and I have intercourse, she says I reach my climax too quickly for her. She says she has timed it to be five or ten minutes, and in this time she is not nearly ready. What is the best thing to do? Also I want sex every night and my wife wishes it only once or twice a week.

Ans. If you carry on intercourse for five to ten minutes, you do it considerably longer than the average man. The average is probably in the vicinity of two minutes, according to the Kinsey studies on the male. You could probably solve the problem if you would prolong foreplay and arouse your wife sufficiently before you engage in intercourse. If your wife begins to gain more satisfaction from intercourse, she might desire it more often. On the other hand, many women seem to be quite content with less frequent intercourse than their husband's desire, even when all is perfect. Some compromise is often necessary.

Fertility Age

Q. Is a woman of 40 or 45 completely fertile? Up until what age can a woman normally have children?

Ans. As long as a woman is menstruating regularly, she may become pregnant. During each menstrual cycle, there is great likelihood that an egg capable of being fertilized is released. The ordinary rule is that a woman cannot be certain that she might not become pregnant until a year has passed without any evidence of menstruation. Of course, fertility begins to decline at about age 35 and is considerably decreased when a woman reaches the age of 45, but there is still a possibility of conception. The average age of menopause, when menstruation completely ceases, is about 49.

Hymen and Virginity

Q. I am unmarried woman, 23 years of age, I am writing to you with the hope that you can clear up some doubts that have been bothering me. I want to know if a young lady is considered to have lost her virginity if a man's fingers have entered her. I hope you understand my problem.

Ans. By definition, a young woman loses her virginity only when a penis is inserted into her vagina. If a finger is inserted, it does not mean that a young girl has lost her virginity. Even if the hymen were ruptured, a young lady may honestly consider herself a virgin.

Blocked Tubes

Q. I have been married seventeen years and I am 34 years old. I have been trying for seventeen years to have a baby and haven't had on yet. So I decided to have X-rays made of my reproductive organs. The X-ray shows that on tube is completely closed & the other is partly closed.

My doctor said he can operate and possibly open the tube that is partly closed, but he can't guarantee that I will have a baby. He said I have a small chance of becoming pregnant. I want to have a baby very much. Do you think it's possible for me to become pregnant?

Ans. Your doctor is quite correct in saying that he cannot guarantee that pregnancy will take place after surgery to open the tubes, but that there is a chance for pregnancy.

It goes without saying that your husband should be examined to be sure that he is fertile. We presume that your doctor has seen to that.

Also where one tube is partially opened it is sometimes helpful for the physician to repeat salpingograms (X-rays), injecting iodized oil into the tubes under moderate pressure. The oil serves to open the adhesions, which block the tube. Where they are repeated two or three times at monthly intervals the tube is frequently forced open. This is much safer and probably more satisfactory than operation.

Superfluous Body Hair

Q. I am 25 years old and my problem is superfluous hair. The hair is on my arms, hands, face and neck. There is no history of anyone in my family having it.

When I became pregnant the hair growth stopped and quite a bit of it even fell out. However, about a month after the baby was born the hair grew back. Is there anything that can be done about it? What might be causing it? I would like to get to the source of the matter.

Ans. Yours is a very unusual case. It would seem that there is some unknown cause for the excessive hair, which is somehow affected by the special hormonal condition of pregnancy. You better consult a competent endocrinologist, who specializes in the various glands and their hormones. You might also be aided by a dermatologist, who specializes in skin disorders.

Cancer

Q. I know it is very rare for women to get cancer of the womb. What happens to their husbands-do they get cancer from intercourse?

Ans. There is no danger of a man's developing cancer if he has intercourse with a woman who has cancer of the womb. Cancer is not a contagious disease, but an abnormal growth of cells in the body.

Maintenance of Potency

Q. I am 43 and my lover is 63. Despite his age and Puritan scruples, I would call him a very sexy man. He is intense, emotional, a poet-and his response to me is immediate. He is also physically very strong, having been a farmer all his life and still doing hard manual work. To me it seems his virility and potency has increased with age, although he takes much longer to reach a climax than I do (which is enjoyable for me). My problem is how to keep him this way.

We now see each other about once a month, since we live at different places. Now we wish to marry. I am thinking in terms of his age and I want to keep him potent and healthy into his eighties. His heart and blood pressure are perfect. Can I, as a younger woman, do anything to keep him potent for a longer time? He has no doubts about himself. He says it is all in your head. I do love him and I want us to continue to enjoy each other for along time to come.

Ans. The best possible prescription for the maintenance of potency in a 63 years old man would be to continue having regular intercourse with someone who reacts towards him, and toward whom he reacts, favorably. You do have to face the fact that marriage sometimes introduces tensions and conflicts that are not present when you are seeing each other only once a month or for an occasional weekend. Being together in the intimacy of marriage does sometimes change things. If however, you can maintain your present attitudes towards each other, his potency could be maintained although some lessening is to be expected.

No one, of course, can know just how long a man's potency will last. In some men it has lasted into the advanced years. There is a very considerable psychological factor, but age does take some toll.

Right Time to Become

Q. I am 22 years of age; I have been married for about a year and a half and so far have had difficulty in becoming pregnant. Could you please tell me how long you should wait before seeing a doctor about this problem? What type of doctor would you suggest I see for this particular type of examination?

Ans. You should make a certain that you have intercourse near the middle of your menstrual month. The twelfth to the fourteenth days after the start of the menstrual flow are usually the days when a woman will conceive. If you do not become pregnant in another six months or so, it would be wise for you to consult a gynecologist. He will want to examine a specimen of your husband's semen in order to determine if his Sperm are normal and present in sufficient numbers. If your husband is fertile, he may want to run a series of tests on you. Sometimes it takes a woman quite some time to become pregnant.

Blood Pressure and Sex

Q. Is there much real danger for a male who has hypertension (high blood pressure) to try and practice a normal sex life? My blood pressure stays around 155/110 and never seems to cause any noticeable ill effects. What kind of sex life would be best prescribed for a person with hypertension?

Ans. A blood pressure of 155/110 is not excessively high and would not seem to rule out normal sexual expression. However, you should seek the guidance of a physician who may give you medication to bring down your pressure somewhat. You do not give us any information as to your weight. If you are overweight, then by all means take some off as that would very much help to bring down your blood pressure.

It probably would be wise for you to indulge in sex activity somewhat circumspectly, that is, without too great emotional tension. But attempting to go without sexual intercourse and, therefore, building up a great deal of nervous tension would probably do far more harm than normal sexual activity.

Hypospadias

Q. I have a condition present ever since birth, called hypospadias. The opening of my penis is along the bottom side of my penis instead of at the tip. Will you advise me as to what should be done for this condition, as far as any possible surgery is concerned? I was told by one doctor, a plastic surgeon, that work should have been done when I was very small. Nevertheless, he thinks the condition I have is not too serious to go for surgery. Is intercourse at all possible with this condition?

Would marriage be a failure with the existing condition?

Ans. Whether or not an operation is necessary or advisable depends entirely upon the degree of hypospadias. In most cases, the urethra is quite normal, running the entire length of the penis, with the opening just at the junction of the shaft of the penis with the corona of the glans. This does not prevent normal erection or normal intercourse. Semen can be deposited in the vagina so the man can father children without great difficulty.

In other cases, the opening is back near the scrotum, which may make it difficult to urinate normally or to deposit semen into the vagina, except by artificial insemination. Perhaps you should consult an urologist, as well as weigh all the factors in your own mind, before deciding whether an operation is necessary. In either event, you should be able to engage in intercourse without surgery.

Masturbation in Females

Q. I am 47 years old and married for 25 years. I have grown-up children. My problem is that I do not fully aroused in intercourse, but get aroused only through masturbation. I have practiced masturbation since I was a girl and I believe it is the reason I fail to respond to intercourse. I have never told my husband or anyone about this habit of mine.

Ans. The most important thing you would need to have in order to learn to reach orgasm through normal intercourse is a cooperative partner. You try intercourse in such a position as to make it easy and comfortable for your husband to stimulate the vulva and the clitoral area very gently during actual intercourse. Once you achieve orgasm this way, even though it was done with manual stimulation, you could ultimately learn to reach orgasm solely through the act of intercourse.

Of course, as long as you go on reaching orgasm through masturbation, you will not build up enough tension to make it easy for you to reach orgasm in intercourse. If you would forego masturbation for a period of time, it might help matters greatly.

Weak Drive

Q. **This question concerns me very much. My age is 24; I have sexual intercourse about once a week with an older woman. I am not married. My problem is that I seldom have the urge for sex. Even with foreplay, I find it hard to get excited. I believe that I lack the sex hormones in the body. Please advise me on this problem, I am deeply concerned because I want to marry and I am afraid I may not be an adequate husband.**

Ans. Perhaps you are not really attracted to your present partner, either because of her age or some other reason. If you were to be strongly attracted to a woman, you might find that you would have very much stronger sexual desires.

Semen As A Laxative

Q. My husband and I have been engaging is oral-genital activity for some time. Now and then I swallow his semen. It is not uncomfortable or unpleasant to me but it seems on me as a laxative the following morning. Is there any danger in that? Is there any evidence that semen has that effect upon people?

Ans. While I have not heard of anyone finding semen a laxative, I can assure you that there is no harm in your swallowing it. There is nothing in semen that would ordinarily cause such a reaction, but we are all different. In any event your have nothing to worry about.

What is A Fetus?

Q. I tuned in the radio the other day on a discussion about abortion, and they were talking about embryos and fetuses. Are those two different words for the same thing, or is there a difference between an embryos and fetus?

And I wonder about another thing, too. How soon after conception is it medically safe for a woman to have an abortion? How is it done?

Ans. The distinction between an embryo and a fetus is time. One source says an embryo becomes a fetus five weeks after conception. However, a current medical dictionary puts the time as eight weeks after conception. The latter time period seems to be more widely accepted.

Most gynecologist feel that it is medically safe to perform an abortion six weeks after conception. It is better to give the fetus a chance to grow a little, and frequently woman will not be sure of pregnancy before six weeks.

When an abortion is done during first three months (12 weeks) of pregnancy, it is usually performed through the vagina. There are two techniques currently being used: a dilatation and curettage (D & C) or by suction. In both instances the mouth of the uterus (cervix) is opened with metal dilators. After the cervix has been dilated, the fetus is either scraped out by an instrument that looks something like a spoon (curette) or by suction.

Self-Gratification

Q. I am 53 years old. I recently started indulging-once or twice a week-in self-gratification, which I find satisfying. Is this practice mentally or physically harmful?

Ans. Medical men today generally agree that self-gratification is not harmful physically. Almost every one engages in the practice at some time in life. If the older tales about it were true, mankind long ago would have perished from the earth.

If one over-indulges in this practice, the potency in intercourse may be lessened, as a result of psychological reasons.

Marriage to Relative

Q. I would like to know whether if I were to marry a second cousin of mine, our children would be abnormal or deformed in any way.

Ans. Marriage to relatives does increase the possibility of passing on bad traits, which might be carried by the genes of both persons involved. In your case, where the relationship is not too close, there would not seem to be much greater risk than in the marriage of unrelated person, particularly if there is no history of serious hereditary disabilities in the families involved.

Breast Surgery

Q. I am professional dancer. I am thinking of having an operation by a plastic surgeon to enlarge my small breasts. Would this new type of operation be conducive to cancer or injurious in any way? I understand a spongy substance is inserted

permanently in the breasts, and then the breasts are sewed up. Could this cause irritation of any sort?

Ans. Medical opinion generally is against the type of surgery you asked about. A method used years ago was the injection of liquid paraffin. Results, usually, were decidededly unpleasant. Just what is conducive to cancer is still doubtful.

Better not have a foreign substance implanted, but consult an endocrinologist. Sometimes small breast are the result of a hormone deficiency.

Small Male Genital

Q. When my wife and I have marital relations she tells me that my genital is so small that she lacks satisfaction. How can the size of my organ be increased? I fear that may wife may leave me because of her dissatisfaction.

Ans. The penis (like the body and its various organs) grows to dimensions according to heredity. Nothing can change this. There is no way by which your male organ can be increased in magnitude-either diameter or length. Dimension, however, is of relatively minor importance, except in the mind of the male who feels that an extremely large organ indicates greater manliness. It does not-many males with large genital organs are sexual weaklings. Learning more about the erotic zones in the male and female should improve your marital relations.

If you change position during intercourse so that your organ will make better contact with the clitoris, you may improve matters considerably and bring about marital satisfaction.

Vaginal Sensation

Q. I have been married four years and have two children. In marital relations, while I almost always reach a climax, I do not sense when the semen is ejected into the vagina. Is something wrong with me? Many of my friends say that they do get this sensation.

Ans. Fewer women then you would imagine actually feel the sensation of ejaculation of the semen into vagina. Many who think that they do actually do not. What they probably feel are the pulsations of the male genital organ when ejaculation occurs. There is much less sensation within the vagina than many believe. The cervix (mouth or neck of the womb) is almost anesthetic (without the sensation of feeling). Many operations can be performed on it without anesthetic and pain is not felt.

There is nothing wrong with you. If you find satisfaction in sexual relation, no more is necessary, and if you are satisfied, you should not worry about your sensation. One's friends are often inaccurate concerning sexual matters.

Injection into Prostate

Q. I have had slight prostate trouble for some time. I am told that there is an infection in the gland. Is direct injections into the prostate gland with antibiotics the best treatment or is it dangerous?

Ans. There is no reason for injection of antibiotic directly into the prostate or any other organ, or gland of the body. We doubt that any well-qualified doctor would resort to such a procedure, except perhaps as an experiment.

Our best advice is that you consult a good and reputable urologist.

Virginity

Q. Does a woman who has practiced self-gratification for many years loss her virginity?

Ans. A person ceases to be a virgin at the time of the first coitus. In the female, an unbroken hymen is generally (falsely) considered a sign of virginity. However, the hymen may be perforated accidentally in a number of ways prior to intercourse. Self-gratification in itself does not affect virginity.

Retarding Climax

Q. In intercourse I reach my climax within a few minutes. I am considering marriage. Is there any drug or prescription I can use to delay ejaculation?

Ans. If you can retard ejaculation "a few minutes" you do not reach your climax more quickly than the average male. You perhaps need no help.

A method developed by doctors, publicized in medical journals and in some magazines, indicates that the application of a mildly anesthetic ointment helps to retard ejaculation. It is applied on the glans penis and surrounding area covered by mucous membrane (not skin). It should be rubbed into the mucous membrane until it disappears. For maximum effect, it should be applied 20 to 30 minutes before engaging in coitus.

Such an ointment may be produced without prescription from drug stores. The ointment is used for numerous purposes and is non injurious.

Masculinizing Tumor

Q. In the last three years I have noticed hair on my face like a man. According to my physician, this is caused by a tumor of the adrenal gland.
If I have this tumor removed, will it definitely cause the hair to leave my face? I would also like to know if this tumor would keep me from becoming pregnant. I have been married fifteen years without children and would like to have a child.

Ans. Of course, the tumor of the adrenal gland should be removed. It endangers health otherwise.
We cannot tell you (nor can any one) whether the facial hair will disappear or whether you may bear children if the tumor is removed. There is a likelihood that the facial hair will disappear. We certainly advise you to have the tumor removed.
Your failure to have children may be due to a number of conditions in either you or your husband. Only a medical examination can determine the exact cause.

Retention of all Semen in the Vagina

Q. My wife and I are anxious to have a child. I have already been examined-the doctor found a high sperm count and good motility.
When does the woman generally ovulate? I notice that my wife, after marital relations, has a habit of urinating. Does she is this way cause a less of semen and thus prevent herself from conceiving? Is it necessary for all the male semen to be retained in the vagina for impregnation to take place?

Ans. Urination on the part of your wife as you described cannot prevent pregnancy. Yet if your wife is anxious to conceive, she should not get up immediately after the marital act. She should lie prone for 15 to 30 minutes with her hips raised. This is routinely done in artificial insemination when the wife has difficulty in conceiving.

All of the semen does not have to remain in the female vagina in order for a woman to become pregnant.

It is considered that a woman ovulates about half way between her menstrual periods, but it is an established fact that a fertile woman may become pregnant at any time.

You should have your wife checked by some good gynecologist. Her tubes may be blocked.

Bosom Obsession

Q. My husband and I have been married many years and have three children. He has always been a good husband and father. He still is very good to me and claims he loves very much, but I have begun to worry about his actions.

He seems to be obsessed with women's breasts, always observing women's figures and making remarks about them. He also kept nude pictures in his workshop until I complained. He doesn't seem to desire going out with any other woman. At night he comes home and spends all his time watching girls on television.

Since I have small breast size his constant remarks about breast size have made me feel inferior and jealous.

Do you think he is satisfied with me, even though he keeps noticing other women? He says he loves me more than ever.

Ans. According to your description your husband may be emotionally immature. It is not because he is not in love with you that he acts as your described.

You also show a lack of maturity in being jealous and disturbed. Ignore his actions and his conduct will improve.
You are needlessly disturbing your-self. He will probably turn to you for love and sexual fulfillment, regardless of these actions.

Pain In testicles

Q. I am 42. At the age of 19, while wrestling, my testicles were subjected to very great pressure. They have hurt me ever since. I am now told by my doctor that to stop them from hurting, I must be operated on to have epithelial cells taken off my testicles. Will this cause me to be sterile?

Ans. We do not wish to reflect on the diagnosis and suggested treatment of any doctor. Perhaps you have not understood his suggestions clearly. We cannot understand how removing "epithelial cells" can help you. Did he say the EPIDIDYMIS? Why not try another doctor-preferably an Urologist?

Pain on Ejaculation

Q. Does self-gratification or intercourse during menstruation cause impotency? Would either of these acts also cause a pain in the genital organ at the time of ejaculation?

Ans. The practice of self-gratification will not cause a pain such as your described in your letter. Neither would intercourse during menstruation.
Nor is impotence caused by either practice. If the pain persists you should consult a urologist. He will not be likely to even, ask you whether you practice

self-gratification. The practice is common and has persisted since long before recorded history. See a urologist and explain that you have pain when you ejaculate. If he asks whether this is during intercourse or at end of self-gratification, tell him. It will make no difference to him-he will probably not be prejudiced.

Climax after Hysterectomy

Q. If a woman has a total hysterectomy, will she still be able to reach a climax during marital relations?

Ans. The female internal organs are not involved in the climax. If the woman has been able to reach her climax prior to the operation through proper marital techniques on the part of her husband and herself, there is no reason why she should not continue to derive complete satisfaction. In some woman, there is even greater satisfaction, since there is no longer any concern about possible conception.

Lack of Sex Drive

Q. **My wife and I have been married for 7 years. Lately my wife does not seem to have desire for marital relations.**
I would like to know if there is some sort of drug or medicine that would stimulate desire for intercourse more often, because our married life is, starting to break up and we need advice.

Ans. There are no drugs that might stimulate your wife's sexual desires. Her lack of desire may be due either to an unfavorable physical condition or to a mental attitude.

We can only advise you to consult a doctor in person to find out if there is a physical ailment. If there is nothing wrong physically, it is necessary to discover and correct any emotional problems, which may prevent your wife from having desire for sex relations.

Diabetes and Impotence

Q. I am 40 years old and my husband is 45. He has diabetes. During the past few months, because his organ will not erect, he finds it difficult to have marital relations, although urgently desiring them. Is this inability normal for a man? What can be done about it? He does not want to consult doctors.

Ans. These are many causes of impotency, such as psychological (10%), physical (85%) and of unknown origin 5%. The cause of your husband's impotence is definitely physical one in origin.

The chief physical causes include the diseases of blood vessels (33%), diabetes mellitus (25%) and endocrine imbalance.

To ascertain which cause is the main culprit please go to the following tests:

1. Blood sugar - fasting and P.P.
2. Testosterone essays, and
3. Penile colour Doppler only on the basis of the above investigations treatment can be initiated.

Effects of Sterilization (Vasectomy)

Q. **i. Will sterilization decrease or abolish the desire for sexual intercourse?**

II. Will it cause sexual weakness in the sex organs and glands?

III. Will it decrease partly or totally the power of full erection?

IV. Will it make more lasting the gratifying sensation in marital relations?

V. Will it cause the ejaculation to be more Easily controlled?

Ans. i. Sterilization will not cause less sexual desire.

ii. Sterilization will not cause weakness of the genital organs, such as the penis, the testicles, the prostate and the lesser auxiliary glands.

iii. Sterilization will not lessen the power of erection. It will not affect erectility in the least.

iv. Will neither lessen nor increase the gratification of sexual relations. It will neither prolong nor shorten the time of the sexual act.

v. Vasectomy would have no effect over ejaculation or ejaculatory control.

Hymen and Virginity

Q. My daughter, as a child while playing had an accident, which ruptured her hymen. Would this be evidence of loss of chastity-even though she is a virgin. Planning to be married soon, she has become self-conscious about it. As a mother, I am interested in guiding and preparing my daughter for marriage.

Ans. Many females are born without a hymen. In many the hymen is destroyed accidentally before the girl child reaches puberty. The hymen is not an evidence of either virginity or lack of virginity. The husband who squabbles with his wife (bride) as to whether she is or a not a virgin deserves neither a bride nor the consideration of decent people.

Orgasm and Nipples

Q. I am a 24-year-old married woman and can achieve orgasm only by having my nipples fondled. Is that abnormal?

Ans. Reaching orgasm by nipples stimulation is not abnormal, but you are in the minority. Sexual research has shown that more than half of all women gain some erotic pleasure from breast stimulation. However, less than three women in a hundred are able to reach orgasm from only this method of arousal.

Male Breasts and Eroticism

Q. Are the breasts, especially the areola and nipple, sexually erotic in men?

Ans. From the point of view of how the breasts are formed and where they are located, the male and female breasts are identical. However, few men like to have their breasts stimulated during sexual intercourse or foreplay. Generally men consider caressing breasts to be a 'feminine activity' and find it either inappropriate or unpleasurable.

Inverted Nipples

Q. My nipples are inverted. Exercises and manipulation have not helped. My doctor recommended surgery. What is the cause of my problem and what type of surgery can be performed?

Ans. Inverted nipples are not rarity. They are due to short ducts that keep the nipple pointing in rather than out. It is a congenital problem; that is, you were born with it. The only effective solution is surgery. The operation consists of cutting small pieces of skin around the nipple and elevating them from the surrounding areola or dark pigmented area, it is not major surgery, and is usually performed by a general surgeon or one specializing in breast surgery.

Unequal Breasts

Q. I am 20 years old and have very small breasts. I would like to undergo plastic surgery to enlarge them. Is the operation dangerous?

Ans. With the new silicone rubber implants, enlargement of the breasts is one of the safest and simplest operations if performed by a competent plastic or breast surgeon. The new breasts look and feel quite normal. The incision is made either under the breast or within the areola, and complications such as bleeding or infection occur in less than two in a hundred women. The implants have been sued for 15-20 years without causing any tumors. Only a tiny scar, if any, will remain.

Q. My left breast is slightly larger and lower than the right. Is there any treatment to make them equal?

Ans. Since the difference in size of your breasts is small, and you have no other abnormality, no treatment is necessary. Your condition is not unique, in fact it is rare to find a woman whose breasts are both exactly the same size (in most people one foot is larger than the other, one arm longer than the other etc)

Sagging Breasts

Q. I am 28 and have breast fed two of my children. Before marriage I had beautiful, large, firm breasts. Now they are flaccid and sagging. How could I have avoided my problem?

Ans. Your problem is very common, and is not related to breast-feeding or size alone it is rather related to unknown individual differences, age, type of skin, weight, size of the breast, and hereditary factors. There is no proven method to prevent the breasts from sagging from childbirth and delivery. Nevertheless, it is believed that proper support during pregnancy and breast-feeding may help minimize the sagging.

Flat Chested

Q. My daughter is 18 and very flat chested. She has become very concerned about and would like to take hormones to increase their size. Is that recommendable? Will she be able to breast feed with her small breasts?

Ans. hormones are not recommended for your daughter's problem. That "remedy" would be worse than the "disease". Many of the devices, hormones, and vitamins that are claimed to increase breast size either do very little or are dangerous. Exercise may improve posture and increase the muscles under the breast, thus giving the appearance of increased fullness.

Small breasts undergo considerable development during pregnancy, but the size of the breast has no influence on the success or failure of nursing.

Pregnancy During Breastfeeding

Q. My baby is three months old and I am breastfeeding. I am not using any birth control method. Can I become pregnant?

Ans. Although breast-feeding may delay menstruation and conception after delivery, it will not prevent you from getting pregnant. Since many women have become pregnant shortly after delivery even before the resumption of normal menstruation therefore it is advisable to use some contraceptive device.

Hair over Areola

Q. I have a few short hair around the areola of my breasts and I am very concerned. What shall I do?

Ans. Women who do not have excessive hair in other parts of their bodies, and whose natural hair is black or brown, often have hair on their nipples. There are several ways of removing them. They could be "plucked" using tweezers, or eliminated by using chemical hair removers or electrolysis. Shaving might lead to more hair growth of a coarser nature.

Extra Nipple

Q. My wife has a "mole" in the right groin and was told by her doctor that it is an extra nipple. Could that be possible? If so, how was it formed?

Ans. Yes, the diagnosis is probably correct. Your wife was born with it. The breast is the first gland derived from the skin to appear when the embryo is around six weeks old. At that time there is a thickening or "milk line" where breast tissue could develop. It goes from the armpit to the groin. This thickening slowly disappears, except in the chest, which later on becomes the breast. Failure of the "milk line" to disappear gives rise to extra breasts or nipples.

Location of Breast Cancer

Q. My friend told me that cancer of the breast does not occur in all parts of the breast with the same frequency. Is she correct?

Ans. Your friend is right. Over half of the time cancer of the is located in the upper part next to the armpit. When you examine your breasts spend extra time in this area.

Breast Cancer in the Males

Q. Do men get breast cancer?

Ans. Men rarely get breast cancer. When they do, it is usually seen after the age of 65, it is 100 times less common than in females.

Heredity and Breast Cancer

Q. My mother and aunt had breast malignancy. Are, my chances of developing the disease higher than ordinary?

Ans. Yes, your chances, are about twice that of a woman without a family history of breast cancer. It is very important for you to examine your breasts monthly, with twice-a-year check-ups by your physician. The need for annual mammography (breast X-rays) should be discussed with your doctor.

Injury and Breast Cancer

Q. I was involved in a car accident and struck my left breast against the steering wheel. A black and blue tender lump developed which slowly disappeared. Will that cause me any problem in the future?

Ans. Trauma to the breasts is common in car accidents, but there is no connection between breast injury and malignancy. Most of the time, the tenderness and colour changes slowly disappear leaving no lasting affects.

Breast Feeding and Cancer

Q. Is it true breast feeding prevent breast malignancy?

Ans. Years ago, it was a common belief among doctors and patients that breast-feeding was associated with a lower incidence of breast tumors. However, the latest research does not confirm that concept. Breast-feeding does not appear to alter the risk of breast malignancy in either the mother or her daughter.

Large Breasts and Cancer

Q. I have always had large breasts. Are my chances any greater of developing a breast tumor?

Ans. There is no relationship between breast size and malignancy. The problem with large breasts is that a small tumor may go undetected for years just because it lies under layers of fat. The smaller the breast, the easier it is to discover small lumps, and abnormalities.

Discharge from Nipple

Q. I am 24, and recently I had a Nervous breakdown. I was placed on large doses of tranquilizers and now I have a white discharge from my nipples. Should I be concerned?

Ans. Milky discharge from the breasts is a side effect of the tranquilizers you are taking.

As the does of tranquilizers is decreased, the milky discharge will also lessen. Has your physician examined your breasts to put your mind at ease.

Pill and Breasts Cancer

Q. I have been taking the birth-control pill for four years with no side effects. Am I more susceptible to breast tumors?

Ans. Thus far, there has been no direct relationship shown between the Pill and breast cancer. Nevertheless, since the pill is nothing more than a combination of small amounts of hormones, Breast Self Examination and an annual check up are recommended.

Cysts in the Breasts

Q. My doctor told me that I have "fibrocystic disease" of the breast and has drained a few cysts. Will they recur?

Ans. Fibrocystic disease is a benign (not malignant) condition found in women. The cysts vary in size from that of a pinhead to a lemon. They make the breasts lumpy and tender. The fluid filled cysts may reappear and will have to be drained again. Fortunately, they tend to disappear after the menopause.

Small Lump in the Breast

Q. I am 20 years old and have found a small lump in my right breast. It is freely mobile and does not hurt. Should I have it removed?

Ans. At your age the most common diagnosis of the lump is a "fibro adenoma". It is a benign (not malignant), painless tumor, and does not become malignant. It should be removed for your own peace of mind—and for a definitive diagnosis.

Mastectomy

Q. What is a mastectomy?

Ans. Mastectomy means removal of the breast. There are several types. In a radical mastectomy, the breast tissue, lymph nodes, and muscles are removed. In a modified radical mastectomy, the chest muscles are left intact but the lymph glands under the arm are removed. A simple mastectomy consists of the removal of breast only.

Tests of Detect Breast Cancer

Q. In addition to breast self-examination what other tests are used to detect breast malignancies?

Ans. The two most common tests are thermography & mammography. Thermography is a method that picks up the heat given off by the breast, translating it into a special photograph. Inflammations and tumors increase the activity of the breast, which is then transmitted through the skin to the special machine. Tumors show up as hot areas. Another technique commonly used is mammography. It uses very small amounts of X-rays to visualize details of breast structure. The radiation dose is very small and has been proven safe.

But in spite of all the latest techniques, breast-self-examination is by far your best weapon against breast diseases.

Tight Foreskin

Q. When I have a full erection, my foreskin retracts as it should, but the sensation isn't very pleasing. It feels very tight. Is circumcision the only solution to my problem? I'd really prefer the alternative if there is a good one.

Ans. The alternative to complete circumcision is a very minor slit in the prepuce; it's called a "dorsal slit". That can be done in the Doctor's office, in a matter of minutes, under a little local anesthetic.

The anesthetic is injected at the top of the prepuce. To visualize that, picture 12 O'clock on a dial. Two small mosquito forceps are then put on the prepuce and a small incision-one quarter to three eights of an inch long-made. The clamps are left on for five or six minutes so that there will be no bleeding and then removed.

You could not have intercourse for several days-five or six at least-until the slits are healed enough so that there would be no danger of bleeding.

The operation would enlarge the opening of the prepuce so that it would then retract without any sense of tightness whatever.

The thing for you to do is to consult a urologist. Be sure you get one who is willing to do a dorsal slit, and who will not insist that the only thing to do is to have a complete circumcision. The latter is totally unnecessary if you do not want it.

Gynecological Examination

Q. Does a doctor, when examining a woman's female organs, insert his hand to her vagina? My wife recently had her first examination of this kind and was under impression that the doctor inserted his entire hand, but after looking at the size of his hands she thought that she must have been mistaken.

Ans. No—the doctor did not insert his hand inside your wife's vagina. Such a procedure would have been unnecessary. Physicians frequently insert a well-lubricated gloved finger to determine whether a diseased or unhealthy condition exists. Frequently the finger is placed against the cervix (neck of the womb) while the doctor's other hand presses on the pelvis. This enables the doctor to determine a number of things about the condition of the womb. When a woman is about to bear a child, doctors may make a similar examination to determine the progress of the baby downward, but at this time the finger usually is inserted into the rectum.

In various examinations and treatments the doctor uses a speculum, an instrument that holds open the vaginal Orifice and the vagina. Various instruments sometimes are inserted through the speculum, some of these being specially lighted to make the internal parts easy to study. The doctor then looks through an eyepiece to determine the condition of the ovaries, the tubes, the womb etc.

Sex and Mumps

Q. I am 23 years old. When I was 16 I had the mumps. As a result I have only one functioning testicle. The other is half the dimension it should be. Would my sex life be affected by this condition?

Ans. A man with one functioning testicle is just as potent (sexually capable and powerful) as a man with two testicles. He is capable of fathering children of both sexes, if the spermatic duct has not become closed. When a man suffers from the inflammation and swelling of the testicles that sometimes accompanies mumps (orchitis) one or both testicles may escape injury; but the spermatic ducts may become closed on account of the inflammation. No way is known whereby this may be corrected.

Should a test be made and no fertilizing elements (spermatozoa) be found in your semen, this would not indicate sexual weakness in any way, but it would demonstrate that you could not become a father.

If you are interested you could have your semen examined to determine whether you are fertile and thus capable of becoming a father. Otherwise you should have no occasion whatsoever for worry.

Menses and Virginity

Q. A women in her forties, whose menses ended four months ago is to be married two months hence, for the first time. Will she react to first intercourse like a young virgin or is there danger of hemorrhage? Could she possibly have a child?

Ans. If the menses have ceased for only four months, no woman can be certain (unless cessation was caused by surgery or X-rays) that she has completed the menopause. If, however, the menopause has been completed, pregnancy cannot take place.

As to how any woman, be she a young virgin or an older virgin, will react to the first intercourse no one can predict. There is far less hemorrhage at the time of first intercourse than is generally believed. Many women do not bleed at all. The Bleeding, if it does occur, seldom is dangerous or anything about which to worry.

Sterility after Abortion

Q. My husband is 39, I am 27, I love my husband very much. It seems that because of an abortion ten months ago, I cannot bear a child. My husband and I are unsuccessfully trying to have a child. Your advice will be appreciated.

Ans. It is possible that you were not injured by the abortion. Consult a gynecologist. He will probably give you some tests to determine whether you fallopian tubes are open or closed. If they are open, you will in time be able to become pregnant. There may be other reasons why you have not conceived. Much can be done today to bring about conception. Your doctor has many means of aiding you.

Fallopian Tube and Pregnancy

Q. My wife became pregnant in her right fallopian tube. Her doctor says that the tube must be removed. What effect will the removal of this tube have on her becoming a mother in the future?

Ans. According to the law of averages, the removal of one fallopian tube will have no appreciable effect in lessening the possibility of a woman becoming pregnant. If the remaining tube is unobstructed, there is probably the same possibility of pregnancy that existed before the removal of one tube.

Large Male Breast Glands

Q. I am 21 years old. My breast glands are larger than normal, causing embarrassment to me. Would it be advisable to have them removed by an operation? Is Homosexuality the cause?

Ans. The condition you described is generally known as gynecomastia. Many males are affected by it. It has nothing to do with homosexuality or with sexual irregularity of any kind. Homosexuality derives from environment and early conditioning. Gynecomastia is a physical condition.

Any good general surgeon can remove the glands mentioned in your letter. Consult a good surgeon. The operation is not dangerous, and a competent surgeon should leave no noticeable scar.

Warts on Scrotum

Q. I have warts or boils on my scrotum. Can you suggest a remedy?

Ans. There is considerable difference between warts and boils. If you have boils, they will soon mature and erupt and healing will occur after drainage has ceased. Evidently you have some form of warty growth.

If you have any form of growth on your scrotum, you should not try to treat yourself. Consult a doctor and let him take care of the condition.

Artificial Insemination

Q. I have been married eighteen months and have not yet become pregnant, although my husband and I want a child very much. He had a sperm

test, which provides his sperm to be healthy. Our marital relations are completely satisfying. We have become interested in artificial insemination or "test tube" babies, but our doctor has completely discouraged us in this respect. We would appreciate information on this subject.

Ans. Possibly you and your husband are too impatient. Many healthy couples do not conceive a child until after several year of marriage.

Conception is something of a chance. You cannot predict when conception will occur. A woman may become pregnant at any time-even while she is menstruating.

Artificial insemination should be used only as a last resort, when all other methods of stimulating or restoring fertility have failed.

I would like to advise you to go to the nearest fertility clinic where every means for assisting you will be available. There are dozens of causes of infertility. The real cause must be determined individually in each case by careful medical study.

Potency after Prostate Gland Removal

Q. If my prostate gland was removed, could I still have satisfactory sex relations with my wife? She says that such an operation would deprive me of satisfaction in intercourse.

Ans. Many men who have undergone surgery for the removal of the prostate gland have remained thoroughly potent after the operation.

If you are potent now, you probably would remain potent after the operation. Sexual potency often is a matter of mind rather than a matter of glands and muscles.

Food and Potency

Q. I am 30 years old and unmarried. I feel that I am impotent. Please inform me as to what kind of food. I should eat to improve my sexual potency.

Ans. The food one eats has nothing to do with potency. In some countries where diets are meager, potency and fertility appear to be great. India and Egypt are examples.

If you believe you are impotent, consult a Sexologist.

Self-Gratification

Q. I have been indulging in self-gratification once or twice a day for the past fifteen years, I am now very nervous and my eyes have set deep in my head. Because of my changed appearance, my fiancée has left me. If I stop this practice, will my eyes remain deep set, or will their appearance again become natural? It is true that self-gratification causes mental disorder?

Ans. The practice of self-gratification does not cause the symptoms you described. The changes in your appearance are due to other causes.

Self-gratification is not a cause of mental illness, although it sometimes is erroneously believed to be responsible.

Evidently you need medical attention. Any good general practitioner should be able to find out what has caused your trouble. Such a doctor will know the best of treating you.

Needless worry and fear concerning the practice can do you harm.

Diabetes

Q. I am 36 years old and I cannot get an erection. Doctors have prescribed hormone shots and several types of pills, but nothing helped. I had a vasectomy to make me sterile about 10 years ago, and I have been a diabetic, regularly taking insulin, for about 7 years. Sometimes I do have an ejaculation but without erection. My marriage has dissolved because of my impotence. What kind of doctor might be able to help me?

Ans. One of the commonest and most bothersome symptoms, which a diabetic can have, is the problem of impotence. We do not really know why this is so. Even when the diabetes is well controlled, there still may be difficulty.

Your vasectomy has nothing to do with your inability to gain erection. The only possible difficulty that could cause would be an emotional one.

I can only suggest that you continue under your diabetic treatment and be sure that you keep it very well controlled. Perhaps you should speak with a psychiatrist, since there is always the possibility that your impotence, which was caused by diabetes, persists because of emotional reasons.

VD Transmission

Q. Can a person get VD through oral-genital contacts? Can the germ be transmitted from genital to mouth as well as by mouth to genital?

Ans. Both syphilis and gonorrhea may be contracted by oral-genital contact. That is to say, if the individual has gonorrhea and the tongue or lips come in contact with some of the germs, it is possible to have a gonorrhea infection of the tongue and mouth.

Syphilis can also be transmitted from mouth to genital. If the individual with syphilis were in the so-called secondary stage, the saliva may be teeming with infective organisms and these could be passed on to the genital and in the same way the germs can reach from genital to mouth.

Excessive Lubrication

Q. When I have intercourse with my husband, there is an excessive flow of vaginal fluid. This compels me to stop and clean myself before we conclude the act. I have tried various douches, which doctors have suggested, but none have been of any help. What can I do the overcome this?

Ans. Occasionally, the Bartholin glands, two glands situated on either side of the entrance to the vagina, do secrete a very considerable amount of mucus under sexual stimulation. If this is the cause of your difficulty, there is no cure short of operation and the removal of one or both of these glands.

The other cause may be cervical erosion. This is a change in the womb neck, which is not cancerous, but does produce a great deal of mucus. To cure it, it is necessary to cauterize or painlessly burn away some tissue from the womb neck. The cure is very simple. It takes about six weeks for a cauterized cervix to heal, but once that is done, the amount of mucus is greatly decreased.

You would have to go to a competent gynecologist and have an adequate examination to see whether or not this might help.

Vaginal Tear

Q. When I gave birth to my daughter the outer part of my vagina was torn. Because of this my husband fails to achieve satisfaction in intercourse. Several doctors have told me that a small operation would cure this. But they also said that if I had any more children the same thing would happen again. I hope to have children. So what can I do?

Ans. If you had a vaginal tear following childbirth this can, of course, be repaired by stitching. It is true that it might tear again with another birth, but in the hands of a skilled obstetrician, using an adequate episiotomies - which involves making a deliberate slit in the vaginal floor and then repairing it-this might be avoided. It is difficult without an examination to give adequate advice. Consult a gynecologist, and be guided by his or her suggestions.

Quick Ejaculation

Q. My case is the following: I am 20 years old and my wife is 23. For the 3 years that we have been married and having relations, I have been unable to bring her to orgasm. I become so excited that I ejaculate almost immediately. This has created quite a bit of tension between us. What can I do?

Ans. You should try to develop techniques in sexual intercourse, which make it possible for you to delay your own orgasm. A variation in position might help, or simply making an effort to relax and not thinking about your impending climax. The important thing is for your wife to reach orgasm. It doesn't matter whether she does it in ordinary intercourse or through caressing and manual stimulation of the vulva and the clitoris.

Some men have reported success with the use of a topical anesthetic ointment. In this country there are at least two brands sold in the drugstore. One is called Nupercainal Ointment and the other xylocaine Ointment. If a little is rubbed into the glans, or the head of the penis, 20 to 30 minutes before intercourse, it sometimes helps to slow up the attainment of orgasm. Occasionally a mild sedative or tranquilizer, taken by mouth, has helped.

Urethral Blood

Q. I am 67 years old. My problem is that for the past few days, after I urinate, there are 3 or 4 drops of blood. I don't feel any pain or irritation. I blame this to over-indulgence. I took my wife to Kathmandu for a week and we drank and played until 4 A.M. and had intercourse every night. Before this we had intercourse 3 times a month. What is your opinion?

Ans. It might well he that having intercourse so frequently did set up an irritation in the back part of the urethra that brought about the bleeding. It may subside without any treatment whatever.

If it persists, or if you have any urinary difficulties you certainly should consult a urologist- a doctor who specializes in disorders of the male sex and urinary organs. Have an adequate examination to find out what the trouble might be and take whatever treatment is advised.

Artificial Insemination

Q. I would like have some information about artificial insemination. Where do they get the semen that

is deposited in the women? Can the woman's husband place it within her or must a doctor do it?

Ans. It is the physician, who places the semen by means of a syringe within the woman's vagina, near the womb. In a few cases the semen of the husband is used. Most often, the semen is obtained from a donor-usually a medical student-who resembles the husband as much as possible. Since the use of frozen sperm has not yet become a widespread practice, semen must be placed in the vagina immediately after ejaculation. The donor is in one room in the physician's office and the patient in another. They never meet or know who the other is.

Cousins Marrying

Q. I am 24 years old and my fiancée is 18. She is a first cousin of mine and our parents object to our marriage, fearing our children will be abnormal. Do you think they are right? We are in love and want very much to marry.

Ans. It is usually considered unwise for first cousins to marry. Many countries have laws prohibiting this. Since first cousins have a common pair of grandparents, if there are any defective traits in them, which have been concealed, there is the possibility that two defective genes might lay opposite each other, and if this were true, a child might very well be born with a serious defect.

Annulment

Q. I would like to know if, in a case where a woman was not questioned prior to marriage as to whether or not she was a virgin, and it turns our she was

not, is the man entitled for annulment. Can he get one on the grounds of fraud?

Ans. Generally, if a woman were not asked about being a virgin before marriage and made no statement to the effect that she was, there would be no case for annulment of the marriage on the ground of a fraud. She had not fraudulently represented anything. She only claimed to be a woman willing to get married and, therefore, there could be no possible question of annulment of the marriage on such a basis. However, a lawyer should be consulted who is familiar with the Indian laws in this connection.

Coital Position

Q. I am 50 years old and I recently married a woman who is 53. It is the second marriage for both of us. We have had many relations during the 6 months we have been married but I am terribly disturbed about one thing. She cannot climax when we are in the man above position. She loses all feeling when we try it. She can climax very fast in the man below or side position. I asked her if the situation was the same with her previous husband, but she evades the question by saying she doesn't remember. Naturally, I can't believe this. She tells me she has never enjoyed relations as much as now. But I feel she says this is not to hurt me. I wonder if my penis could be smaller than her deceased husband's. I do feel terribly inadequate and puny because I can't make her respond normally. My penis is 7" long when erect & 1-5/8" in diameter. Do I compare very unfavorably with other men?

Ans. When two people have been married previously, there is sometimes an emotional problem. Where there have been years of sexual association with another person, a pattern has developed which may be difficult to change.

Your wife very possibly got into the habit of having sexual intercourse in the women above position with her first husband. They might have been very satisfied with that position and, therefore, she has developed the habit of doing it that way. She may learn with you if you are both patient to do it in the man above position. It is true many women prefer the woman above position, because it enables them to control their movement and have clitoral contract. There is no harm in letting her reach orgasm in the woman above position and then reverse the position so that you can go ahead to reach orgasm and gain complete satisfaction in the position that is most satisfactory to you.

Your penis at 7 inches long and 1-5/8 in diameter is definitely above the average, so you should have no concern about the question of the size of your penis giving complete satisfaction, although penis size has really little or no importance in successful sex functioning.

Virginity

Q. I am 23 years old and will soon marry. When I was quite young I fell over an iron her fence and was taken to the hospital because I was bleeding from my vagina. I recall that the doctors inserted instruments into my vagina.

I forgot about this until recently when I realized that because of this I can no longer be considered a virgin. I am very uneasy that my future husband will make an issue over this. Can't I still consider myself a virgin?

Ans. A girl is a virgin until she has had actual sexual intercourse. Only when a penis has been introduced into the vagina is the girl considered no longer a virgin. If you had an accident, which made examination of the vagina necessary, it may be true that the hymen has been destroyed, but the fact remains that you are still a virgin girl if you have not actually had sexual intercourse.

Your husband should realize that at least 30 per cent or so of all young women do not bleed at first intercourse even if there has not been any accident that might have destroyed the hymen.

Alcohol

Q. I am 28 years old and married. My wife and I are very anxious to know if a child will be abnormal if it was conceived under the influence of alcohol.

Ans. A child would ordinarily not be abnormal if it were conceived while one or both partners had had a considerable amount of alcohol. This would not affect the sperm or egg of the parents or the child's development in the womb.

Breast Pain

Q. I am 45 years old. My breasts are large and they pain me. The doctor told me that I suffer from chronic cystic mastitis I have no idea what that is. What is it and can it be cured?

Ans. Cystic mastitis is an inflammation of the breasts due to cysts, which have developed within them. The administration of some progesterone hormone sometimes helps in such cases, though your doctor must decide if this advisable on the basis of having examined you thoroughly. Sometimes an operation to remove the Cysts, which create the discomfort, is the only solution.

Male Sterilization

Q. As I understand the male sterilization operation, called vasectomy, is foolproof. If the sperm tubes are cut and tied off, or if a segment of the tubes are removed, how could sperm possibly get into the ejaculate? Nonetheless, I have been told by people that the operation isn't always successful. They say that women have become pregnant even after their husbands operated upon. How could this be?

Ans. You do have to realize that mistakes can be made and the physician might think he had cut a portion of the sperm ducts, when actually he had gotten a blood vessel, or something of the kind, so that the individual was not sterilized. There is always the possibility of having a double duct on one side so that if the surgeon did get one, but did not get the other, sterilization would not be complete. Naturally, he would not be searching for both, since this is relatively very rare. The possibility of the rejoining of the duct following even a successful vasectomy does have to be considered. All of these possibilities are very rare.

Following a successful vasectomy there are still sperm in the seminal vesicles. Not until the individual has ejaculated some 10 to 12 times and then brings in a specimen to be examined under a microscope to make sure that there are no sperm present can a man be sure that he is completely sterile.

Safe Days

Q. Which days are the safe days for a woman to have sexual intercourse without fear of pregnancy? If one counts the days correctly, is this method absolutely reliable?

Ans. The so-called safe days are usually from the beginning of menstruation until the 9th day following the start of menstruation. The 10th to 15th days following the start of menstruation are the days when most women would become pregnant if they had intercourse without contraception. After the 15th day a woman is not very likely to become pregnant until the 10 day following the start of the next menstruation again. However, there are many exceptions to this general pattern and women have been known to become pregnant from intercourse during the so-called infertile days. The "safe" days also depend on the length of the woman's menstrual cycle and on her regularity. Therefore, the "safe" days are not absolutely safe.

Masturbation

Q. I am 45 years old and single. Sometimes I indulge in masturbation, doing it at bedtime. Then I become nervous and cannot fall asleep. I have tried masturbating until the point of orgasm and then stopping. However, I have been told that doing this is even worse than completing the act. Is that true?

I have also been told that wine mixed with an egg, or orange juice with an egg and a few drops of lemon juice, is very good for sexual vigor. Is that true too?

Ans. Your nervousness following masturbation is undoubtedly due to your emotional attitude towards it. If you could accept masturbation as perfectly normal and beneficial where it relieves sexual tension, you would really have good sleep following it.

It is true that stimulation to the point of almost reaching orgasm and then stopping leaves a prostatic and rear urethral congestion that is definitely worse than going on to orgasm, which brings about the relief of this congestion.

It has long been thought that consumption of raw eggs, either in orange juice or wine may help improve one's sexual vigor. It is only due probably to the fact that the individual is then having a high protein diet. Certainly there is no harm in it, and if it seems to help, if even on a psychological basis, it might be worth trying. Actually, an adequate diet is all that is necessary to maintain sexual vigor. Special foods probably exert any influence they may have by their psychological effect.

Frequent Urination

Q. A year ago I contracted a venereal disease. I immediately saw a doctor who cured me within a matter of 2 days using penicillin. However, ever since then I have had to urinate very frequently. I returned to the doctor and he gave me douches of my urinary passage and he also massaged my prostate. These treatments haven't helped and I am wondering what else I could do?

Ans. You should consult a urologist, a specialist in disease of the genito-urinary tract in the male. You might still have an infection of the prostate. You might also have an inflammation of the urinary canal. It is possible that you have a small closure of the urinary passage and an instrument should be passed in the urethra to find out whether or not this is so. Certainly in competent medical hands, you should be able to be cured without much difficulty and in a reasonable period of time.

Tight Prepuce

Q. My 6-year-old son's foreskin is so tight that it permanently covers the head of the penis and can never be pulled back. The boy suffers pain when his penis becomes erect. I am sure that smegma secretion is accumulating beneath the foreskin too.

My wife and child live in Bombay and my wife opposes circumcision on religious grounds. I think that for hygienic reasons the boy should be circumcised. What is your opinion?

Ans. If your son is suffering from a prepuce so tight that it causes difficulty, he certainly should be circumcised. Complete circumcision, of course is not exactly necessary. A small slit can be made through the prepuce permitting it to be retracted. This is a very simple operation that could be done under a little local anesthetic. Perhaps, if you approached a doctor with the idea of doing a slit rather than a complete circumcision, it would solve your problems and you might gain your wife's consent to have this done. Certainly it could be important for the health of your son.

Q. I have been a paraplegic, paralyzed below the waist, for 2 years now. However, I still have erections and there seems to be ejaculations. Is it possible for me to have offspring in my condition? I am 25 years of age.

Ans. If you can have erection and if you can have an ejaculation, you could, of course, impregnate your wife and very possibly have children. One man we know was almost completely paralyzed, and had to live in an iron lung for many years, but during that time he fathered 3 children.

One Testicle

Q. I had an undescended testicle removed years ago, and so I only have one in my scrotum. Even though my marriage is a happy one, and I have a 3-year old daughter, but having only one testicle has always affected me. I always had a complex about this. Can anything be done?

Ans. You are overly concerned about having only one testicle. That fact that you have been able to father a child is adequate testimony that you are not infertile. If, however, it means a very great deal to you to have a normal appearing scrotum with two testicles in it, a competent urologic surgeon very possibly could and would be willing to put in a prosthesis, which would make your scrotum appear normal. By all means call a hospital and get the name of 2 or 3 urologists to whom they will refer you, one of whom you can choose to consult.

Masturbation in Marriage

Q. My wife and I have been married 18 years. We have intercourse 3 to 4 times a week. We have found that about once a month we prefer mutual masturbation. We don't want to use anything that would harm ourselves. Do marriage counselors consider that there is anything wrong in this?

Ans. Generally, marriage counselors believe that any form of sex play is acceptable which the couple finds mutually agreeable. The couple themselves must make the decision about which is "right" and "wrong".

Cysts on Scrotum

Q. On my scrotum there are many little growths that look like pimples. When I squeeze them pus mixed with a little blood comes out. My skin is generally greasy. What can be done about this condition?

Ans. You undoubtedly have several little so-called sebaceous cysts. The best possible thing for you to do is to consult a dermatologist or possibly a urologist, and then be guided by his suggestion as to treatment. Bathing in good hot water, sitting in the tub for 10 to 15 minutes, will frequently make it possible to easily evacuate these by a gentle squeezing. But you should have expert advice on the basis of an adequate examination.

Quick Ejaculation

Q. My husband always completes intercourse before I reach climax. We have a tried various position as well as lengthy foreplay, but he can never control himself. Is there anything else he could possibly do to help himself?

Ans. Some men have found it useful to purchase a tube of Nupercainal or Xylocaine ointment, either of which can be obtained at any good drug store. If a little of this is rubbed into the glans, or the head of the penis twenty to thirty minutes before intercourse, it will commonly make it possible to delay orgasm for several to many minutes.

In some cases, counselling is needed to clear up an emotional problem.

Sterilization

Q. I am 27 years of age. I have already had three children and I am now pregnant with another. Would you please give me some information about having my fallopian tubes cut to prevent future pregnancies. Is it safe?

Ans. Since you have three children with a Fourth soon to be born, there is no reason whatever why you should not have your tubes tied. In a hospital there is a rule that any woman who has had as many as three children is entitled to have her tubes ligated if she wishes to have this done. There is no untoward sequel that is likely to follow so long as the operation is performed by a competent surgeon. It is done about the third day after the baby is born and it might mean that you would have to stay in the hospital an additional two or three days, but if everything went entirely satisfactorily it would mean no more than that.

Ovarian Tumors

Q. Will you please tell me what causes tumors? I have had two fibroid tumors removed and I now have an ovarian tumor.

Ans. One of the mysteries of modern medicine and surgery is just what causes benign tumors. Inheritance plays a large part. If your mother had uterine fibroids, then you may inherit that tendency.

If you now do have an ovarian tumor, and if it is large enough to be giving you any difficulty whatever, it would undoubtedly be wise to consult a surgeon about its removal.

Closed Fallopian Tubes

Q. **I want very much to have a child but I am unable because my fallopian tubes are closed. I don't know how this came about and I don't know what can be done about it. Will you advise me?**

Ans. It would be impossible for us even to guess as to what might have caused your fallopian tubes to be closed. If you have had any vaginal infection or have had a miscarriage or abortion, this might have introduced enough infection into the womb to account for it.

The only thing for you to do is to put yourself in the hands of a very competent gynecologist. He can run tests to find out whether or not your tubes are open. If they are closed, it is sometimes possible to perform an operation that would open them. This, however, would be a moderately costly procedure with the surgeon's and the hospital bill. But that is unquestionably the best possible advice that we could give you.

Female Sex Satisfaction

Q. **In recent issue of some magazine, a woman doctor was quoted as saying that it is not necessary for the husband to have an erection in order for wives to enjoy sexual relations. What did she mean by this?**

Ans. The doctor was referring to the fact that it is, of course, possible for the husband to stimulate the vulva and the clitoris in other ways sufficiently to bring about orgasm in the wife when it is impossible, for any reason, for him to have an erection and carry on intercourse.

Disproportion in Size

Q. **My age is seventeen and wife is eighteen. Whenever we have marital relations, I feel that she's not getting full satisfaction even though she has never mentioned it. My wife's vaginal passage is rather large. I would also like to know if there is any way to make the penis larger?**

Ans. Since you are only seventeen, if you would consult a competent sexologist, it might be possible to give you some hormone injections that would increase the size of the penis, if it has not reached full maturity.

Diabetic's Sex Problem

Q. **My friend confided her marital difficulties to me. Her, husband, who is 48 years old and a diabetic, is sometimes very lovable and desirous, while at other times, he is cold. He never has a full erection and he comes to a climax too suddenly, which leaves her unsatisfied. I think it is because of diabetes, but she fears it's because he doesn't care for her. Isn't it harmful to her to never be satisfied?**

Ans. It is true that diabetes in a male frequently brings about the condition known as impotence or the inability to have an erection sufficient to permit intercourse. His mental and emotional attitude towards that may contribute to his percipate orgasm so that she does not have time to reach a climax and gain release from sexual tension herself. The one thing that could be done, of course, would be for him to continue stimulation of the vulva and clitoris, if necessary, to be sure that she has the opportunity of gaining the release from sexual tension, which she should.

Morning Erections

Q. I am 27 years old, single, and enjoy good health, but I do not have morning erection as other men do. Does this signify some infirmity or lack of potency?

Ans. The fact that you do not have morning erection may be of no significance whatever. You give us no information as to your potency when attempting intercourse. If you are able to carry on intercourse in a satisfactory manner, then of course there is absolutely nothing about which you need have the least concern.

Semen Absorption

Q. I am unable to have intercourse because of a sick wife. Does semen 'cake up' in the body when ejaculation does not take place. Also, the glans head is dry and wrinkled. What can be done about it?

Ans. Semen does not 'cake' in the body or anything of the kind. When it is not ejaculated, some may be reabsorbed.

If the glans seems unduly dry, the best possible thing to do would be to put a little Vaseline, cold cream or bland ointment of any kind on it. This would soften the mucous membrane of the glans and prevent its drying out to such a degree.

Female Breasts

Q. I have several questions. First of all, what is a gynecologists? Also, why do some women have large breasts and others tiny ones? What can be done to prevent large breasts from being pendulous and drooping?

Ans. A gynecologist is a physician specializing in the treatment of women, especially the reproduction organs. The size of the breast on a woman is not only a matter of the fat, which she has on her body but also of course, to an extent, it is heredity. That is to say, you may have breasts similar in size of those of your mother or your father's mother.

An adequate breast support, well designed to keep the breast up, preventing them from hanging down and stretching out the little fibrous bands that support the breasts, is advisable in cases of pendulous breasts.

Late Pregnancy

Q. I am 53 years old, married, and I have two grown sons. I stopped menstruating two years ago. However, I underwent tonsil operation less than a year ago, after which I menstruated once and haven't again since that time. Is there any danger now that I may become pregnant?

Ans. While, as one might say, nothing is impossible, it would be most improbable that there would be any danger of a woman becoming pregnant at the age of fifty-three when she has not menstruated for so long a period.

Hairiness and Sex Desires

Q. Does the hair covering on legs, arms, armpits and sexual organs indicate sexual potency of individuals? Does heavy hair growth indicate more potency sexually? What are 'signs' of sexual potency that doctors look for in a person? Does voice, speech, body movements indicate anything in regard to sex ability?

I've noticed some loss of hair on my legs. Does this mean I am losing a certain amount of sexual desire (I am 35)?

Ans. Although certain types of hair growth are secondary sex characteristics, which appear when the sex glands mature, heavy hair growth does not indicate greater sex potency. Loss of hair would in no way be a sign that you are losing sex desire. Men who have lost all their body hair due to a disease called alopecia have not been affected in their libido.

The secondary sex characteristics - hair, voice, body changes, etc - may sometimes indicate to a physician that something is radically wrong with a person's glands. In the normal person such features would in no way reveal the individual's sex desires or capacities. These are generally determined by early experience and psychological factors as well as by physical makeup.

Frequency of Sex Relations

Q. I have heard many women say that they have marital relations only once or twice a week. Others say they have sex relations daily. Which is the most favorable frequency in marriage?

Ans. There is no frequency which is 'most favorable' or preferable. Each husband and wife must work out their own pattern of sexual life, based upon their mutual desires, needs, capabilities and habits. Some couples may be satisfied with relations occurring once in several weeks; others may desire such relations more than once daily. The important thing is that the frequency should be mutually satisfactory.

Fatherhood Test

Q. Can the blood of a baby and its supposed father be compared in order to determine if the father is really the parent of the child?

Ans. In the case of the male, negative parenthood is the only thing that can be established. That is, if the supposed father and the child are not in the same blood group, the man cannot be the father. If the baby and the suspected father are in the same blood group, the suspected male may be the father.

Childlessness

Q. I am 27 years old and my wife is 24. Though married five years, we have no children. A test has shown that my sperm count is satisfactory. Tests have shown that my wife's oviducts are open and that no spermatozoa were alive thirty minutes after marital relations.

Ans. We believe that there may be an insufficient amount of HYALURONIDASE (an enzyme or ferment) in your ejaculate to penetrate the tough coating of the ova (eggs) of your wife to permit fertilization. But she may at any time produce ova, which have a less tough covering. Patience and time are, therefore imperative.

Repairing Enlarged Vagina

Q. I am 31 years old and my wife is 26. We have been married for eight years and have two children. Our sex life was normal until our second child was born four years ago. Since that time my wife has had difficulty in attaining satisfaction from marital relations. Her vagina is larger than it was before the last baby was born. She says that my organ is not large enough and that she therefore does not experience any gratification. She cannot reach a climax and her ungratified desires leave her frustrated.

Ans. The enlarged condition described in your letter is one that is quite common after childbirth. During the birth of a child there is considerable pressure against the tissues and often serious tears occur. The attending physician usually sews up these latter. Now and then even an observant doctor will not notice some of these tears. Often very small tears occur. Under favorable condition these heal and the parts return to normal size. When they fail to heal properly, a weakened and enlarged channel results.

The condition can be readily corrected by surgery that is not dangerous or serious. It is a simple operation usually performed at the surgeon's office.

Gonorrhea Test

Q. How can one tell whether a woman has gonorrhea?

Ans. There is but one actual way to tell whether a woman has gonorrhea, and that is to have a physician take a vaginal smear, make a slide and do a microscopic examination. Even this may have to be repeated for absolute certainty. There are no dependable symptomatic signs. While women with gonorrhea often have itching in the vaginal tract and some discharge or burning on urination, these symptoms are no certain indication of the disease.

Trichomoniasis

Q. I just had a pelvic examination and the doctor said I had an infection called trichomoniasis. I'd like to know what causes this and whether it is dangerous? Can I become pregnant while I have this infection?

Ans. The cause of the infection you have is a tiny parasite, know as the trichomonad. The condition is uncomfortable and contagious but not dangerous. It has nothing to do with whether or not you can become pregnant. But your doctor should treat it.

The disease is spread in a number of ways. Your husband should be examined too; otherwise there is constant danger of husband and wife reinfecting each other.

Gynecomastia

Q. I am 26 years old and for the last five or six years my breasts have been gradually enlarging. They are not so large as to be noticeable when I have a dress shirt on, but are large enough to be noticeable if I wear only an undershirt. I am ashamed to take my shirt off in public because they look like the breasts of a young woman. I am not fat but have always been rather on the skinny side. I have been putting on weight recently and my breasts are more evident than before.

What causes this condition? Of more concern to me is what can be done about it short of surgery? Is this an indication of homosexuality?

Ans. Your condition as described in your letter positively is not an indication of homosexuality. Homosexuality is not a physical condition.

You should lose no time in consulting an endocrinologist. Enlargement of male breasts, or gynecomastia, is caused by a number of physical disorders. Medical treatment will depend on the physician's diagnosis of its cause.

Replacing Organs

Q. About seven weeks ago I was pregnant in one of my fallopian tubes. I had to have surgery and my womb and tubes were removed. Please tell me if they can be replaced. It seems now that almost any kind of surgery can be performed and I want to have children more than anything in this world. I'm 26 years old and have one son age 8 years.

Ans. Surgery cannot replace your organs, which were removed. Our advice is that you will find greater peace of mind by devoting yourself to the child you now have, and perhaps, by adopting others.

Insensitive Clitoris

Q. I would like to have a few questions answered about a woman's clitoris. My wife claims she has no sexual response to stimulation of the clitoris. I would like to know what is the cause of this, and if in any way it could be restored to its proper functioning again.

Ans. Your wife may be suffering from sexual anesthesia, or lack of gratifying sensations. Every case is a law unto itself. The best solution that we can offer is a through examination by a gynecologist. There are innumerable possible causes in such cases. The only way that you can learn of the possibilities, one way or another, is through the findings of the examining gynecologist. A possible cause may be a hooded clitoris. The hormone testosterone has in some cases been helpful in increasing erotic sensitivity of the clitoris.

Lack of Lubrication

Q. I am 48 years of age. I had my uterus removed about fifteen years ago. I remarried a year ago. When we have marital relations, there is no moisture in the vagina, and it is very painful, often leaving me sore for a day or so afterwards. I very seldom come to a climax, due, I think to the pain of intromission. However, I can come to a climax by self-gratification.

Is there anything that can be done to correct the above situation? I have my ovaries, and have not had an examination since I have remarried.

Ans. Perhaps your glands of Bartholin are inactive. These are two tiny pinkish glands situated one on each side, just inside the vagina. You might ask a doctor to examine these glands. They function in sexual excitation and furnish lubrication. In such cases, both husband and wife applying a good lubricating jelly can relieve the pain of intromission. A neutral jelly doctor's favourite is K.Y., and this is obtainable at practically all drug stores. A prescription is not needed. Your problem should readily be solved through cooperation of both your husband and yourself.

Climax in Pregnancy

Q. Does climax in intercourse cause any harm when one is five months pregnant? Could it cause premature birth?

Ans. Reaching a climax does not cause harm in pregnancy. Dr. Alan Guttmacher, one of the best known experts in the field, has said: "it is in no way harmful for a woman to experience orgasm during pregnancy; actually, its achievement is just as beneficial and important as at any other time."

In cases of women who habitually miscarry, or where a miscarriage threatens, physicians often prohibit intercourse altogether during pregnancy.

Pubic Hair Growth

Q. I would like to ask at what age would the growth of pubic hair be definitely expected. My son is well past fourteen but as yet has no visible growth of pubic hair. He is well developed otherwise. Most of his close friends now have a growth of pubic hair and also of hair under the arms, and of course he is becoming quite self-conscious about the matter. Could it be that some boys do not start developing hair until well into their last teens? What should I tell him?

Ans. It is possibly somewhat unusual for your son to have reached the age of fourteen and still have no visible growth of pubic hair. However, there is no need to be too concerned about it for at least another two years. If by the time he is sixteen, he has not shown some growth of pubic or an armpit hair, then you should take him to a physician for a competent examination. But at this time it is advisable to wait for some time.

Sterilization Effects

Q. What are the effects of a sterilization operation in a woman? How many days must elapse before sex

relations can be resumed? Might the first coitus after the operation be painful?

Ans. A sterilization operation with the cutting and tying of the fallopian tubes has no effect upon a woman sexually. She would feel quite normal and her sex desire should not be lessened in any way.

There is no reason to feel that first coitus after the operation would be painful. Of course, since the operation requires an incision in the abdominal wall, it might well be three or four weeks before a woman could engage in intercourse in any satisfactory fashion following such an operation.

Female Pubic Hair

Q. I am wondering whether it is wrong to allow the pubic hair to grow long. Isn't this unsanitary, in that it would be easy for germs to breed?

Ans. It is ordinarily far better for a young woman to let the pubic hair grow quite naturally. We have never seen a case where the pubic hair becomes so long that it could possibly cause any trouble.

Penile Dimensions

Q. I have observed that some men's genital organs are somewhat more larger when flaccid as they are when they are tumescent. What is the explanation for this?

Ans. In some cases the cavernous, or hollow portions of the penis may be somewhat more fibrotic (containing a large amount of fibrous tissue), and therefore, they do not subside as completely when the penis is flaccid as in other cases. This makes the penis appear almost as larger when soft as when erect. In the average normal case, of course, this is not so. It should also be pointed out that size of the flaccid organ has little significance.

Pre-Coital Douche

Q. Both my wife and I have been married previously, but we have a rather unusual problem. My wife is in the habit of douching prior to sexual activity. She also refuses to engage in any petting or foreplay before coitus. Because of vaginal dryness, intromission is not possible without the use of a lubricant (Vaseline) which both of us find unsatisfactory.

Ans. Taking a douche just before sex relation removes all the normal secretions from the vagina and makes it dry. Taking a bath before intercourse is of course quite permissible, but a douche is not advisable since it interferes with normal sensation.

Vaseline does inhibit sensation since it is something of a foreign lubricant. Certainly it is much better to engage in some preliminary sexual play. When sexual arousal takes place, the vagina becomes lubricated by its glands. If a lubricant is desired. K.Y. Jelly would be suitable.

Breast Surgery

Q. I am the mother of three children and am 32 years old. My breasts are large and I would like to have surgery done on them. They are terribly flabby and have a lot of fatty tissue. Do give me some advice as to whether I could undergo this operation without harming my health.

Ans. Some twenty years ago operations on the breasts had a very considerable vogue. Then came the reaction to them and it was found that, while the breasts could be made smaller and could be made to stay up more firmly, it was very difficult to maintain a smooth soft contour. The interference with the blood supply of the fatty tissues of the breast would make the breasts appear lumpy and uneven in many cases, and this became worse with time.

You might consult a competent plastic surgeon and be guided by his suggestions. He would know whether or not something could be done and yield a reasonably satisfactory result.

Such an operation is not injurious to health and if it could be done, there would be no reason to anticipate any great difficulty.

Prostatitis

Q. I am 24 years old. Three years ago I began to feel an itch in the urethra. Sometime before I had had gonorrhea, but I think I was cured.

The itch is stronger now and after urinating, I have a milky secretion. Several doctors have told me it is urethritis, but I did not get any relief from their treatments.

My doctor says I have prostatitis and I am prone to have orchitis. Another doctor (Homeopathy) says the swelling of the testicle has nothing to do with my prostatic condition. Who is right?

The doctor has prohibited all sex relations. I am very fearful because I plan to marry very soon.

Ans. From your description of your condition it seems that you may have a prostatitis. In the presence of a prostatitis it is not unusual for the individual also to develop an epididymitis. The epididymitis is a part of the vas just where it begins as a tightly coiled, very tiny tube just above the testicles. The prostatitis certainly can contribute to and possibly cause the orchitis or epididymitis.

In the presence of prostatitis, whether or not the individual should indulge in sex relations is a moot question. In some cases it seems to aggravate the condition and in other it seems to help. Only your own personal experience will help to solve that problem.

All means, try to find a very competent urologist and put yourself in his hands and be guided by what he tells you to do by way of treatment.

Ovarian Removal

Q. After 6 years of marriage I was operated upon for a hemorrhagic cyst on my right ovary. Both the cyst and the ovary were removed as well as another cyst on the left ovary. I now have only a portion of the left ovary. Is it possible for me to have a family?

Ans. While the chances of your becoming pregnant are rather slight, no one can say that it is impossible. So long as there is any normal ovarian tissue left and so long as the fallopian tubes are in good condition, it is possible for a woman to become pregnant.

Wedding Plans

Q. I am planning to marry soon. The date schedule for the wedding is 2 days after my menstrual period stop. Is there any chance that I could become pregnant on my wedding night? Would it be harmful to take the contraceptive pills in advance of the wedding?

Ans. If you are to marry 2 days after your menstruation is over, the chance of your becoming pregnant just then would, of course, be minimal although it is not absolutely impossible. The most fertile time is generally around 12 days after the period begins, or approximately 7 or 8 days after it ends.

On the other hand, if you wish to use the birth control pills, you must start taking them before you are to be married. As your doctor will explain to you, you count the first day of menstruation as one and on the fifth day, you start the tablets. You take the tablets for 21 days, then you stop taking them and within 3 days you will menstruate. Again you count that first day of menstruation as one and on the fifth day again start the tablets. If you keep up that up very faithfully you can be reasonably sure that you will not become pregnant until you wish to and discontinue taking the tablets.

Penis Enlargers

Q. I want some expert information about those devices that are advertised as penis enlargers. I thought this was impossible, but they make this claim.

Ans. There are no devices, which will enlarge the penis, despite their claims. There are some types of vacuum pump devices, which will, of course, draw blood into the penis and even over-extend it.

These devices are definitely dangerous. They may bring about a fibrous de-generation of the cavernous spaces of the penis and do real harm.

The size of the penis is a hereditary matter. If it is undersized because of some hormonal difficulty and this is treated during the teenage period, possibly then the penis size may be brought up to normal size for that individual. But it is impossible to increase the size of the penis once the individual has passed the period of youth.

Dryness of Vagina

Q. **I am 28 years old and my husband is 37. We have been married for 5 years. I have a problem that may cause me to lose my husband, if I don't do something about it. It seems that my vagina is dry and I am not able to secrete fluid. I went to my doctor, but he dismissed me by saying I am too young to have such a problem. I was too embarrassed to ask any more questions. Please tell me what I can do? My doctor examined me, said there is nothing wrong and I am in good health. Obviously there is something wrong.**

Ans. It might be very helpful for you to obtain a vaginal cream containing estrogen, a female sex hormone. It is available with all the leading chemist.

If this were applied to the walls of the vagina for 3 or 4 days, and then at the rate of twice a week, it ought to increase the tone of the vagina and bring about a normal output of mucus secretions. It is true, as your doctor said, that most women do not encounter this difficulty until after the menopause when the ovaries cease producing large amounts of female sex hormones. However, some younger women do have this difficulty too. You might discuss our suggestion with your doctor and see whether he agrees that this might be a helpful course.

Impotence

Q. **My age is 48 and I have been impotent for the past 3 years. This state has put me almost out of**

my mind, not to mention my wife's condition. The need and desire for sexual intercourse is present, but the ability is gone.

I am extremely sensitive and embarrassed about this condition and have not been able to consult a doctor because of the embarrassment. I must do something because I feel very useless. Can hormone injections help me? If I do see a doctor what type should it be?

Ans. You should have no feeling of embarrassment about consulting a physician over your difficulty with impotence. It is an everyday occurrence for a competent sexologist or an urologist to deal with such a problem.

It is possible that some testosterone (male sex hormone) injections might help. It is too bad that you have let the whole situation go on for as long as 3 years. That may complicate adequate treatment. You must realize that there may be some physiological cause for it such as, for instance, diabetes, which makes you impotent. If that were corrected, the situation might be changed.

It would probably be better to consult a sexologist although a good urologist would be able to deal with the problem also. If they can find no physical cause, psychological help might be the next step.

Condoms

Q. The use of rubber condoms is the birth-control method my husband and I would prefer to use. However, I have been told that contact with the rubber and chemicals that go into its manufacture can cause cancer for the woman. Is this true?

Ans. The use of a rubber condom certainly would not cause cancer. You should put your mind completely at rest on that score. It is nonsense.

Obstructed Tubes

Q. I have been married for almost 3 years and have been unable to become pregnant. This is because my fallopian tubes are obstructed. I have had 10 insufflations in which air has been blown into my tubes, but they did no good. The doctor says I must have an operation. Can the operation help? Is there any other kind of treatment that might be successful? My husband has had sperm tests and he is a normally fertile man.

Ans. Before having an operation because of tubal obstruction, it would be wise to have salpingograms made. This means injecting an iodized oil solution through the womb and into the tubes to determine where the obstruction may be. It is similar to the tubal insufflations excepting that instead of being done with air or carbon dioxide, it is done with an iodized solution. The iodized solution sometimes opens the obstruction.

The operations for obstructed tubes are very delicate and are very often unsuccessful.

Aging Effects

Q. I am 67 years old. At one time my penis was 7 inches long. Now it is only 4 ½ inches. Can you tell me the cause of this? It also has a curvature now.

Ans. A curvature is often due to what is called "Peyronie's Disease." This is the formation of an inflammatory area in the spongy tissue of the penis. You should consult an urologist and get his advice on the basis of the adequate examination.

The decrease in size of the penis may be simply due to age, since you are 67 years old. Again, the urologist might be able to help you. The change in the penis tissue may account for it also. There are some diseases, which occur very rarely, involving general demasculinization including shrinkage of the penis, but most probably it is a change, which is due to ageing and possibly lack of use of the organ.

Tube Operation

Q. After 2 cesarean births, at the insistence of my husband I permitted doctor to tie off my fallopian tubes to prevent future pregnancies. Following that we divorced and now I am married again.
My new husband wishes to have children so I returned to the doctor. He untied one of the tubes-the other he believed impossible to save-and put a catheter inside it for 4 days to keep it open. Both my ovaries are in perfect condition, though, I have a fibroid tumor in my womb. He thinks I have a good chance of becoming pregnant. Do you think it's true?

Ans. Because you have had both tubes operated upon for sterilization and then had one reoperated trying to restore fertility, the possibilities of your getting pregnant are very greatly reduced.
The fact that you have fibroid in the womb also militates against the possibility of your becoming pregnant. It is impossible to say that you cannot become pregnant, but the possibility of your doing so is certainly relatively small.

Pre-Coital Muscus

Q. I've been dating a wonderful girl for about a year. Since I've been dating her, I've had no sexual

experience with her or with any other girl. I masturbate about 4 times a month. Do you think this is too often?

When I'm with my girl I get an erection very easily. When I get the slightest bit sexually aroused I secrete a clear liquid from my urethra. Is this normal? Is there any way to prevent it?

Ans. Masturbation 4 times a month is certainly not excessive. Whatever frequency you desire, as long as it does not become an all-consuming preoccupation, is perfectly all right. The secretion you speak about comes from tiny glands in the urethra. It is perfectly normal. In some individuals is far more profuse than in others. Practically speaking, there is no way of controlling it other than to avoid sexual excitement. The purpose of it is to lubricate the urethra and to alkalinize it to permit the passage and survival of sperm in the semen at the time of orgasm and ejaculation.

Becoming Pregnant

Q. I am a recently married woman, 36 years of age; I have had no luck in my attempts to become pregnant. I never reach orgasm at the same time as my husband. Could this be the reason I don't become pregnant?

Ans. It is not necessary for you to reach orgasm to become pregnant whether or not you reach orgasm at the same time as your husband, is not in the least important. For emotional reasons, it is important that you should reach orgasm, but this is not essential for pregnancy.

You should go to a competent physician and have both yourself and your husband examined. The starting point is with him. He should be examined first. If he is normally fertile, then it is time enough to start examining you, which is much more complicated. If there is nothing the matter with you vaginally and if your womb is in a normal position, then you must consult a competent gynecologist who will take X-rays of the tubes. This will show him whether or not your tubes are open. He can also determine if you ovulate-release eggs-normally.

Amount of Semen

Q. What can cause a lessened amount of semen to be ejaculated at intercourse? Is excessive work, or perhaps a slight cold responsible? Could it be caused by too frequent intercourse?

Ans. If intercourse is had very frequently, the amount of ejaculate will be markedly decreased.

Excessive work or a simple cold or other minor health trouble would not have a significant effect.

Spermatorrhoea

Q. I am 21 years old. For two years I have been suffering from a dangerous disease. I have consulted several doctors, but in vain. I pass a drop of semen every morning before urinating. Nocturnal emissions occur regularly about every third night. I pass watery semen. My sex organ is very small and not strong. If I married in this condition, how would marriage affect me? Could I regain my lost energy and acquire health again?

Ans. It is perfectly healthy and natural that one or more drops of clear (sometimes slightly cloudy or milky) fluid should be observed at the external outlet of the male urethra) on arising in the morning. This is as healthy and natural as the morning erections experienced by most males.

Nocturnal emissions (except when a number of such emissions occur every night as a result of inflammation or some other disturbance) are in no way unhealthy or injurious. Indeed, in the male who does not have occasional intercourse or participate sexually in some other way leading to climax, nocturnal emissions are a sign of healthy sexual state.

The size of your genital is of little consequence-probably none. The semen of all males sometimes appears somewhat watery or diluted. The seminal fluid of your nocturnal emissions (in your sleep) may have quite a different appearance.

You need no prescription and, as far as your letter indicates all you do need is to give up fear and worry and live according to your most natural inclinations. I am sure, if you would marry there would be no problem and your married life would be successful and happier. So go ahead.

"Old Wives' Tales"

Q. I have heard stories of women having given birth to puppies or partly human and partly animal offspring. Is it possible for animals to impregnate human females?

Ans. Hybridization of cross species has occurred between various animals and insects, but there is not one authentic case of crossing human species with any other species not even apes or monkeys.

Most of these "Old wives' tales" are ridiculous This as you probably know, is impossible. Even prenatal thoughts (a woman's thoughts and habits, etc.) Have no influence over what a child will be-all of this be carried in the genes (hereditary factors) when pregnancy took place.

Impotence

Q. I am 61 years old and apparently am becoming impotent. In the marital act my attempts are often unsuccessful and unsatisfactory. Would "Spanish fly" improve me sexually?

Ans. It is advisable for you to see a competent sexologist. Your letter does not indicate that your diminished potency is necessarily due to a disease or a physical condition. The latter includes age.

The drug "Spanish fly" or cantharides is not an aphrodisiac; it is dangerous and poisonous and has never contributed to the potency either of man or the lower animals. I am sure in the hands of a competent sexologist you would regain your lost potency.

Colored Semen

Q. During the past six months, I have often indulged in self-gratification. I have not had sexual relations for almost a year. I have noticed recently that my semen contains a rust-colored substance. I work in an automobile body paint shop.

Ans. Probably the condition you described has nothing direct to do with self-gratification or ejaculation, but the condition may result from some industrial condition to which you are susceptible.

Consult an uro-sexologist who will analyze the specimen and find out the reason for the discoloration.

Low Potency

Q. I am a married man 39 years of age and have been married for the past twelve years. I have

two children and I consider myself to be in fair health.

My problem is in regard to sexual intercourse. At the present time I average about once per month with my wife. I would like to have more frequent relations but do not seem to be potent more often. I work on a job that has three shifts and every week I work on a different shift. Could this have an effect on me?

Can you prescribe any kind of vitamin tablets for me that would help me overcome this matter and increase my potency?

Ans. If your potency is all right on the occasion when you do have sex acts, then the problem at other time could be caused by some physical factor such as fatigue, or a psychological factor such as worry, anxiety etc.

On the other hand, there are many persons who, for constitutional reasons, are able to have sex relations only infrequently. If your infrequency does not create a problem between you and your wife, you need no help to increase your potency. Your job may possibly have an effect by creating fatigue or anxiety or by its irregular hours. But if your wife is not satisfied by your performance.

It would be a good idea to have a thorough physical check-up to see whether any physical cause is present which is responsible for the condition.

Coitus after Childbirth

Q. I expect to be delivered of my first child in the near future. Since I have heard conflicting reports, I am wondering whether sex relations are in any way changed after childbirth.

Ans. Gynecologist report that, as a general rule, coitus after childbirth is more satisfactory for both partners than it was before. Sometimes, when marital relations are first resumed intromission may prove difficult because of tightness of the vaginal opening, due to scarring from the incision which the obstetrician may have made to prevent tearing during labor. This, however, is usually only temporary. Many women find that they experience a climax for the first time following the birth of a child.

Spinal Injury

Q. I am 24 years of age. Two years ago an injury to my spine resulted in immediate paralysis of the lower half of my body. During the past two years I have recovered considerably but although erection is attained normally, I am unable to reach climax during sexual intercourse.

I have hopes of getting married soon but before I do I would like to know if anyone has regained his sexual abilities after such an injury and what are my chances of being able to father children in the future?

Ans. Only time and experience can determine your future sexual abilities. The amount of sex impairment would depend on the extent of nerve injury and the extent of recovery. You should by no means give up hope.

If you are fertile and can ejaculate during intercourse you can father children.

In order to know whether or not you are fertile you will have to have your semen tested by a physician.

Men who have been paralyzed have been able to father children and engage successfully in marital relations, depending on the specific nature of their injury.

Possible Conception

Q. If after marital relations during which contraceptives are used, marital relations are again entered into a second time shortly thereafter, is it possible for a woman to become pregnant if no devices are used the second time?
Several friends said they became pregnant this way and I wonder whether the male, which would cause conception, would retain some slight amount of semen.

Ans. It is quite possible for a woman to be impregnated during a second intercourse following the first by a short period of time.
In the first place, sperm may be retained on the organ or in the urethral passage from the first occasion, and secondly sufficient sperm may still be present in the male seminal vesicles to cause fertilization after a second ejaculation.

Pregnancy Signs

Q. What are the first signs of a woman's being pregnant and how many days after impregnation do the signs start to show up?

Ans. A woman first suspects that she is pregnant when she misses a menstrual period. After that, signs develop rapidly. The vaginal lips and the area around the nipples become darker and the breasts and abdomen begin to enlarge. Morning sickness with vomitus occurs, but less frequently than in the past. Frequency of urination is common, as well as lassitude and changes in appetite.
When there is doubt, a physician should be asked to make a pregnancy test.

Angularity of the Penis

Q. I am 21 years old and have been married for a short time. When my organ becomes erect, it bends at a considerable angle. What is the cause of this? Also, what can be done to correct it? Is it serious? I have read sex manuals but have never seen any information on this.

Ans. Angularity of the penis is so common that perhaps the majority of men experience it in some degree. Many mistakenly believe that it is due to self-gratification. It is not. It is due to the fact that not all parts or organs of our bodies develop equally.

If the angularity of your penis does not interfere with marital relations, you have no cause for worry. If there is serious interference, plastic surgery to equalize the hollow bodies of your penis can correct the condition, if an urologist feels it necessary.

Unusual Semen Colour

Q. For the last two months, I have noticed that my semen has had a trace of red in it, which might be blood.

My health has been excellent during all the time. I would like to know if the change in colour indicates a dangerous condition.

Ans. We have had many letters from men who complained of the appearance of a red tinge or color in their semen. The condition may result from numerous causes such as infection, injury. We usually advise with such complaint to consult an urologist.

Minimum Size

Q. A doctor told me that to have satisfying sexual relations for both male and female the male organ has to be at least five inches in tumescence. Could a person with a shorter organ expect any kind of satisfaction for himself and his wife?

Ans. Regardless of measurements a sex organ, which erects and remains erect for the sexual act, is entirely adequate for both male and female. It is by no means right to think that five inches is a minimum. Actually doctors have reported satisfactory sex relations in males whose organs had been amputated, leaving no more than one-half an inch.

You should not worry about your size, but learn as much as possible about marital techniques from an authoritative book on the subject.

Lack of Hair

Q. My problem is that I have very little pubic hair and no under-arm hair at all.

I am married, twenty years old and have three children. I feel too embarrassed to talk to a doctor about my condition. I've been to doctors while pregnant but they never mentioned anything about it.

The nurses in the hospitals do, which makes me feel awfully embarrassed. Would anything help my condition or can it be corrected?

Ans. Your condition is nothing about which you should be in the least embarrassed. As a matter of fact, many women remove the hair from under their arms for cosmetic reasons. And there are some women who remove the hair from the pubic area also.

Every physician has encountered women who had no pubic hair at all. This means that there must be vast number of them. An endocrinologist could tell you whether the lack of hair is connected with any abnormality of development or glandular deficiency.

Hymen

Q. **I married when I was 31 years old. I had not sexual relations with any man, also had not engaged in self-gratification. My mind always occupied otherwise.**
My problem is that my husband is not certain of my virginity. He says that when a girl marries at this age, her hymen should be tough and difficult to penetrate and that she should hemorrhage instead of bleeding a few drops. Please advise me.

Ans. If your husband consults any medical expert on this problem, he will find that his belief is altogether wrong. There is no general rule that the hymen of a woman of your age is tough and resistant & hemorrhage is always present. Women differ in these as in all other respects. In addition hymen is not the proof of virginity. In some women it is absent at birth, in others it is broken accidentally during early years. Your husband seems very foolish indeed to allow suspicions based on ignorance to spoil your marriage.

Varicose Veins

Q. What causes the veins on the sides of the penis to become enlarged and varicose? Can this be corrected by surgery or other medical treatment? What would cause the scrotum to hang loosely below and away from the testicles?

Ans. Varicose veins result from many causes. They occur most commonly in the legs, but are also found in other parts of the body. Of course they sometimes occur on the penis. Surgery is of little avail in cases such as that described by you. Nature promptly establishes new blood paths. Varicose veins result from broken down valves within these blood vessels.

Your description of the scrotum indicates a condition, which is quite natural and quite common. Occasionally it requires correction by surgery.

Coital Frequency

Q. What should be the usual rate of frequency of marital relations between married couples? When does rate of frequency become harmful?

What effect does frequency of sex intercourse have on the health and longevity of the average male? This is in relation of the fact that women live longer than men.

Ans. There is no "usual" rate of frequency that should be observed. Couples vary greatly in their desires, needs and abilities. It is up to each couple to decide for themselves what is best and most desirable for them. No one else should be considered. Frequency rarely becomes physically harmful because nature will call a halt, particularly in the male.

As far as anybody knows, the frequency of sexual relations is not related to longevity, either in the case of the male or female. Longevity depends basically on inherited factors. The fact that women live longer than men is due to other factors than sex relations.

Stretching the Penis

Q. I would like to know if I could enlarge and lengthen my penis by pulling it gently several times a day. This is the way that members of some African Tribes enlarge their lips. One thing worries me. Could this stretching of my penis be harmful?

Ans. Stretching your penis will not enlarge or lengthen it. If you are over 21 or 22 you have passed your period of growth. Nothing can be done after this period to enlarge your penis.

Stretching your penis could be harmful. I strongly urge you not to do it.

Strengthening the Vagina

Q. I am 32, married, and have two children. Recently, my husband has come to prefer anal intercourse. It is not very appealing to me; I wonder why he doesn't like regular intercourse anymore. I do not mind anal intercourse once in a while, but I wish he would desire sex in the usual way. Could there be something wrong with me?

Ans. If your vagina had been torn during childbirth, or has become considerably looser, this could explain why your husband now prefers anal intercourse. Your anus would now be much tighter and thus give him more pleasure.

I recommend that you have an examination to see if your vagina was torn. If it was, then it could be repaired by a vaginal plastic operation.

If there is no damage to your vagina, then you should practice exercise to tighten up your vaginal muscles. You should squeeze your vaginal muscles as hard as you can, and hold the tight for about a minute. Do this 12 to 15 times a day.

Within a few weeks you should find yourself gaining a great deal of vaginal control. Continue the exercises for a few months. You should then have enough control over your vaginal muscles so that you can squeeze his penis with your vagina during your regular intercourse. That will give him a great deal of pleasure. Chances are that he will not insist upon anal intercourse very often after that.

There may also be a psychological reason for a man preferring anal intercourse.

Pregnant Virgin

Q. I am 26 and expect to marry soon. My girl and I have petted heavily, but we have never had intercourse. I know she is a virgin because I have felt her hymen.

Her menstrual cycle has been fairly regular for the past two years 28 to 30 days. Last month she started menstruating on the 35th day and had a full period. But this month she has not started her period and it's now the 38th day.

Is it possible for a woman to become pregnant without intercourse? Could there be any other reason for her period being so later?

Ans. If you have indulged in heavy petting to the point where you ejaculated near her vulva, then she could have become pregnant. This does not happen often, but it is known to happen. A girl's hymen has small holes through which menstrual blood and vaginal secretions can flow. A little semen could enter her vagina through one of these holes. There could easily be enough sperm in that tiny quantity so that one can reach the ovum. Only one is needed to fertilize an ovum.

It is possible that her hormones have become unbalanced due to fear of pregnancy. That could cause a delay in her period. I would advise her to see a physician for examination. If she is not pregnant, hormones might produce a menstrual cycle.

Infidelity Check

Q. My husband is in the Navy and almost finished with a two-month cruise. A friend of mine said that there are ways to tell if a man has had intercourse during a short period like this. She didn't explain, and seemed embarrassed when she found out that I did not understand her.
Is there some physical indication, which could show me whether or not my husband had intercourse while he was away? I am not really worried because I trust him. But now I'm curious.

Ans. Your friend is mistaken. The only way a wife could tell whether her husband had intercourse during a two-months absence might be if he returned with VD. Otherwise, there are no physical symptoms, which would indicate that he's had intercourse.

"Let Down" Feeling

Q. I have seen it stated in many places that masturbation does not harm a man's potency. But I have found from experience that it give me a "let-down" feeling.
One thing I wonder about: Can prolonged masturbation get a person so used to self-stimulation that he could not perform competently in marriage? I know of two cases where married men could not have an orgasm without resorting to rapid manual manipulation of the penis.

Also, if a person is in the secondary stage of syphilis, can he transmit the disease?

Ans. There is an old Latin saying, which translated, reads: "All animals feel depressed after coitus." The let-down" feeling is merely a sense of relaxation. One has been tremendously stimulated; now all the tension is gone. That is perfectly normal and is not harmful. Orgasm habits-such as the habit of reaching climax through masturbation-are not easy to change. But they can be changed through re-education. A man who is used to reaching orgasm through rapid manual stimulation of the penis will have to learn to respond to slower motions, s well as from the different sensations, that vaginal stimulation provides.
There are visible symptoms of secondary-stage syphilis—eruption of the skin. Even inside the mouth. At this point, the disease is easily transmitted to one's partner during sexual intercourse or other close contact, such as kissing. The third stage of syphilis is the one in which symptoms are not apparent, although the disease can still be transmitted to one's sexual partner.

Blood Appears in Semen

Q. What could be the cause of red smudges in my semen? Could it be blood? They appear in the more solid parts of my ejaculate. Is this caused by too-frequent sex play, or might it be the symptom of some other condition?

Ans. Without a careful examination, it would be impossible for me to say what is causing blood to appear in your semen. If a small vein toward the back of your urethra bursts at the time of orgasm that could account for it. Stones in the prostate could also be a cause.

I can only suggest that you consult an urologist for an examination. The chances are that you have no real reason for worry, but it would be better to check out the situation. That would put your mind at rest.

Origin of Sperm

Q. I am 47 and have been married since I was 20. My wife and I have always had a satisfactory sexual relationship, but I am curious about one thing. Except for four or five times in my life, I have always felt the semen come from one of my testicles when I ejaculate. Twice, I have felt it come from both at once. Is this sensation common?

Ans. Just what sensation you get that makes you feel your ejaculate is coming from one testicle or both at once is difficult to explain. The point is that ejaculated semen does not come from the testicles at all.

It comes from the seminal vesicles and the prostate, both of which are deep in your pelvis. At the time of orgasm this area goes into spasms, which result in the semen being expelled from the penis very forcefully.

Sperms are constantly flowing from your testicles into your seminal vesicles, but it would be impossible for any man to ejaculate directly from his testicles.

Sagging Breasts

Q. My wife is 50 and her breasts are baggy and nipples very large. Will any sort of medicine shrink the breasts and nipples, or is there an operation that would do it?

Ans. Operation to make large or sagging breasts smaller were very popular 25 to 30 years ago. But such operations have lost popularity because some women experienced uncomfortable side effects. There is no medicine a woman can take that will shrink the breasts and nipples. I suggest consulting a plastic surgeon and see what he advises.

Rectal Itch

Q. For about five years now, I have frequently been bothered by a rectal itch. It usually comes on during the summer. I have been treated by our family physician, but he could not help me. He referred me to a skin specialist, who helped a little - the itching was eased for a short while.
Do you think that an urologist could help me? If not, what sort of specialist would you recommend?

Ans. A physician who specializes in treating diseases of the anus and rectum would be better for you than an urologist. You should consult a proctologist.
You should have a through examination made of your stool to find out if there are any bowel parasites that might be causing your difficulty. The fecal matter needs to be examined several times before the presence of parasites can be determined.

Most Fertile Days

Q. I am 23 and have been married several years. I have never been pregnant. Can you tell me what is the best time of the month for conception?
Sometimes my menstrual period starts on the 8th day of the month, sometimes the 9th, and sometimes not until 12th. How can I figure out my most fertile time?

Ans. We consider the 13th day after the start of menstruation as the most fertile one. Count the day your period starts as day 1 then plan to have intercourse on day 13. Do not have intercourse for four days before day 13, and then on your target day, have intercourse twice. The second act of coitus should follow the first as quickly as your husband can manage.

If you do not conceive the first month, then consider the 12th day as your target day the following month. If this fails, try the 14-day the next month, the 15th the month after and the 10th the next month. This is the usual programme that is recommended when pregnancy is desired and the couples are known to be fertile.

Your most fertile day should be one of those mentioned above. If none of them works out then I advise a fertility examination by your physician for the both of you and your husband.

Worried about Bent Penis

Q. I am 21. I have masturbated since I was 12. I think that has caused my penis to bend to the left, although it is only noticeable when erect. I know it cannot be cured-but is there any possibility of my having intercourse with a girl?

Ans. There is nothing unusual or abnormal about a man's erect penis bending somewhat to the left or right. It is very frequent, and never caused by masturbation. The penis contains "hollow bodies" on the left and right sides. When you are sexually stimulated in any way, these hollow bodies fill with blood. That is what makes your penis swell and become stiff. It often happens that the hollow bodies on one side of a man's penis are smaller than on the other side. As a result, when both fill with blood, the larger side will become thicker than the smaller side; the penis will then bend in the direction of the bigger side.

That condition will not cause any trouble in intercourse. When your penis is inserted into a woman's vagina, the walls, of the vagina expand to accommodate it. The vagina is very flexible and can easily adjust to a large penis or a bent one.

So, if you will merely stop worrying about having injured yourself, you should not have any difficulty in intercourse. Your penis would still bend as it does even if you had never masturbated in your life.

Unwanted Hair

Q. I am 24. I have excessive hair on my legs, and now I'm getting it on my arms. What could be the cause of it? What can I do about it?

Ans. Usually, the amount of hair on a woman's arms and legs is a matter of heredity. Your mother, or one of your grandmothers, had this condition and you have inherited the characteristic. If this is the cause, then nothing can be done about it.

Sometimes, a change in the hormones that come from the ovaries results in greater hair growth. You might consult an endocrinologist to see if he thinks that is the cause. If it is, hormone treatments might help.

Shaving the lower legs, as many women do, can take care of that problem. It is better not to shave the arms, unless the hair is tremendously excessive. The other methods for removing hair are waxing, bleaching or use of depilatories.

Sexual Atheletes

Q. I am 27and single. I enjoy intercourse, but I cannot continue once I have had an ejaculation. Am I sexually inferior? I have heard that most young men can have relations three, or four, or even five times a night. But no matter how long I abstain, I lose all my desire with one ejaculation.

Lately I have noticed clear lumps in my semen. That worries me. Are they a sign of something wrong?

Ans. Even man experiences what is known as a refractory period after ejaculation. Until period passes, he cannot obtain another erection. It may last a few minutes in some men, or several hours in others.

The important thing is whether you have a feeling of satisfaction and completion after you ejaculate-not how often in one night you can do it. It is true that some men are what is called a "sexual athlete," and can reach orgasm several times a night. But the average young man finds that reaching orgasm once satisfies him. There is certainly nothing wrong with you so long as you are satisfied. It is very foolish to expect that you be able to keep up with some other man.

Semen is frequently lumpy. If put into a container and allowed to stand for 15 to 20 minutes, it turns into a clear non-lumpy liquid.

Impotent at 48

Q. My husband is 48. For the past two years he has been completely impotent. We have been married for 27 years, and once had good sex relations. He is a good, kind, considerate man, but his inability to perform is destroying both of us.

He had some hormone shots from an urologist a year ago, but they did not help. The doctor told him that his trouble was mental, not physical.

I can make myself as attractive as possible, but nothing seems to arouse him. He says he has no sexual desire at all-not even for another woman. Is there any way of getting my husband back to normal? My own desires are reaching the point where I am thinking about relations with another man. But I don't want another man; I want my husband as he used to be.

Ans. Has your husband had a complete medical check-up? If he is either diabetic or pre-diabetic, there could be a physical cause for his trouble. Such a condition may seriously affect a man's sexual ability.

His problem seems to be more a lack of desire than actual impotence. That very possibly could be due to emotional causes rather than physical, as the urologist said.

If a thorough examination does not reveal any physical cause, then the thing for your husband to do is consult a trained counsellor, such as a psychologist or psychiatrist. He must be willing to work through his emotional problems, if these are the roots of his trouble; and he will need your help, too. If he is to be cured, you will have to work out the problem together.

Seven-Inch Penis

Q. I am 23 years old and think my penis is not of normal size. I have problems satisfying some girls. When I am erect, my penis is only seven inches long, and four inches long when limp.

Is my penis large enough? What is the normal size for satisfying a woman? Can anything be done for me, which will make penis larger?

Ans. Since we consider five to six inches the normal size of an erect penis, you need not worry about yours being small. It is actually one inch above the normal. So far as size goes, you are perfectly capable of satisfying a woman sexually.

The size of your penis is only a small part of the picture. Since your is neither abnormally large or small, you must take into consideration emotional matters. Loving attention, consideration, thoughtfulness, and the extent of foreplay a woman needs are very important. Also remember to prolong intercourse long enough so that your partner can reach orgasm and thus, sexual satisfaction.

VD Anxiety

Q. I have a vaginal discharge and am afraid that I may have picked up VD. How can I find out for sure? How can I get treated for it? Will I be able to douche while I'm being treated? Should I see a gynecologist or some other special kind of doctor?

Ans. A gynecologist can determine whether or not you have VD and give you the proper treatment for it. If you have any suspicions about having VD, you should not delay having a through examination.

However, the fact that you have a vaginal discharge does not necessarily mean that you have VD. There are other more likely causes, such as yeast infection (monilia) or trichomonas. Cervical erosion may also produce a discharge. All can be treated successfully.

Making Childbirth Possible

Q. I am writing to ask you about the possibility of my wife becoming pregnant. I understand that if a

woman's Fallopian tubes have been cut, then there is no chance of pregnancy. But if they have only been tied, it may be possible for her to have a baby. She had an operation affecting her Fallopian tubes; I want to know if her fertility can be restored.

Ans. When a woman is sterilized, the Fallopian tubes are both cut and tied. Whether your wife's fertility could be restored would depend upon how much and what part of the tubes had been cut away.

Only the doctor who operated upon her could give you a reliable answer to your question. It is possible to restore a woman's tubes to normal after they have been cut or tied, but the chances of success are often small.

Intercourse Time

Q. How long does each act of sexual intercourse last?

Ans. There is no set time, it can last a minute or an hour. It also depends if you count love play (foreplay) as part of the sexual intercourse or only as a preliminary. The only statistics that exist refer to the time that it usually takes for the partners to reach a climax, or orgasm. In men this is about three to nine minutes, in women about five to ten minutes but there are wide variations. After male orgasm has occurred sexual intercourse is soon over, for the man loses his erection. But then you might count any caressing or kissing following intercourse as also being part of sexual intercourse itself.

Sexual Advances

Q. Would you say that is always up to the man to make the first sexual advance?

Ans. Only in Victorian Novels! These days it might be either the man or the woman who makes the first advances and probably this has always been so. What happens in theory in sexual matters is very variable in practice and anyway what is a sexual advance? Surely it can be a smile, a squeeze of a little finger, or even a sigh.

Love Bites

Q. What are love bites exactly?

Ans. They are marks made by the teeth on somebody else's skin in the heat of passion. Sucking another person's skin can also produce bruise marks known as love bites. Oddly perhaps we human are not the only animals to bite one another during sexual excitement. Horses and some birds do it, for example.

Bites that actually break the skin (they many bleed or a little oozing is evident) are potentially quite worrying as even the cleanest teeth and mouth are swarming with all sorts of germs which are quite harmless where they are (in the mouth) but can be infectious when introduced into the skin. If the bite gets sore or nasty looking see a doctor.

Knowing S.T.D.1

Q. How would I know if I had caught a sexually transmitted disease (STD)?

Ans. Men can usually tell quite easily because they get a discharge from the penis or develop a sore or growth on the penis. Some women get a discharge, pain on passing water, or a sore or unusual growth on the skin around the opening to the vagina. But a discharge in women may be nothing to with STD and in many cases the girl who has caught this notices nothing wrong at all.

If anyone is any doubt a check up can be made in confidence, at any special clinic. Ask for the special clinic or the STD clinic. Your family doctor will also advise you.

Oral Sex

Q. What is meant by oral sex?

Ans. Oral refers to the mouth and so oral sex means contact between the mouth and the primary sexual organs-the penis or the perineum. The perineum is medical word used to describe the area between the legs starting with the pubic hair in the front and extending to the anus (back passage) at the rear. Oral sex, therefore, involves sucking or kissing the sexual organs of the other. When a couple do it to each other at the same time it is often referred to as "position 69".

Masturbation: Defined

Q. What is meant by the words masturbation and mutual masturbation?

Ans. Masturbation comes, like most medical words, from the Latin and means" do defile by the hand". This tells us what our forefathers (and mothers) thought of masturbation! Mutual in this sense means "done by each towards or with regard to the other", which gives a good idea of what the mutual side of masturbation is all about. We can forget about the "defiling" bit and substitute the words "giving pleasure" instead. And so mutual masturbation becomes giving pleasure to or with regard to the other, usually with the hands.

Masturbation by oneself is giving pleasure (for its own sake or as a release from sexual tension) to oneself- usually with the hands, so in practice mutual masturbation means he or she giving sexual pleasure to either one of them or more often to both of them (mutually). Usually hands used on the sex organs is the way that people masturbate but not always. Some couples devise other ways of pleasuring one another sexually. Mutual Masturbation is often used to induce orgasm in one or both partners without sexual intercourse taking place. It does nobody any harm.

Wet Dreams

Q. What is a "wet dream"?

Ans. It is a sexual dream that results in a man having an ejaculation of semen either during the dream or shortly after waking. The content of the dream may be only mildly sexual. Wet dreams are entirely normal and do not lead to any illness, weakness, or disease; neither are they indicative that the dreamer is over sexed or lecherous. In all probability they are part and parcel of the male sexual apparatus "running itself in". Usually the dreams completely disappear once regular sexual intercourse (or masturbation) is the normal way of things.

French Kiss

Q. What is French Kissing?

Ans. French kissing is open-mouthed kissing (as opposed to kissing on the lips or cheeks) in which tongues are mutually used to give oral (mouth) pleasure.

Anal Sex

Q. What is anal sex and is it safe?

Ans. Anal sexual intercourse, in which the penis or sometimes the fingers or hand are introduced into the anus (back passage), is certainly not safe. AIDS and infective hepatitis, together with other sexually transmitted diseases, are spread in this way. Furthermore anal sex is illegal under the age of 21 and in some other circumstances (such as the Armed Forces).

Sex in Standing Position

Q. Can one have sex standing up?

Ans. Yes, it is possible to have sex in a wide variety of ways but standing up is by no means the most comfortable or enjoyable method. An old wives' tale used to say that if a girl had sex standing up she would not get pregnant. Many girls have become pregnant unwittingly by believing this fallacy.

Sex and Weakness

Q. Is it "weakening" to have a lot of sex? If not, why do athletes and sportsmen avoid sex some days before the event?

Ans. No, it is not weakening in any way. Sportsmen usually do what their trainer tells them to do and most trainers play it safe in every possible way when giving advice to their athletes. Some top athletes freely admit that they regularly have sex the night before an event and claim this improves their athletic performance enormously'.

Sex Aids

Q. Do sex Aids help people with sex problems or is they for amusement only?

Ans. Sex aids fall into various categories. Female masturbation devices (vibrators and dildos). Vibrators are devices, often penis-sized or penis-shaped, containing a battery which activates a small electrical mechanism that makes the whole aid shake or tremble at high frequency when it is switched on. Women use them to stimulate the clitoris or vulva or more rarely the vagina in which case the vibrator is eased in an out of the vagina. Some sex therapists recommend the use of vibrators for women who are having difficulty with sexual arousal or orgasm. Dildos are solid non-mechanical artificial penises in various sizes made of rubber, vulcanite, or wax. Some are elaborately designed. Occasionally over enthusiastic use causes damage to the entrance to the vagina. Although used mainly by women for self or partner stimulation, some men and women use vibrators and dildos in their love play. Both devices have certain uses for the sexually disabled.

Male devices used to stimulate the clitoris. These are rings usually made of latex that fit around the base of the erect penis. Attached to the ring is some sort of "stimulating device"-maybe a pad or air cushion or soft rubber "spiky" projection. The theory is that during intercourse the woman gets extra stimulation when the man wears these devices. Few women find the use of such devices acceptable or pleasurable or in any way necessary. Most people consider them fun objects. Sprays, cream, and lotions. Many types exist. Their names, with a variety of tantalizing trade names, indicate what they hope to offer customers. Invariably results are disappointing. There are also local anesthetics, designed to blunt the mucous membrane of the penis, which claim to prolong intercourse. Usually they do not work and incidentally have the same effect on the female sexual mucous membrane. They have no place in helping people with sex problems.

ARTIFICIAL VAGINAS: These male masturbation aids are sometimes called a "sailor's sweetheart". They come either as an entity on their own or are part of a "blow-up" female doll. Some of the latter devices are manufactured with a similar artificial mouth and rectum for simulated oral and anal sex. They are generally unhelpful for those with sex problems but may be a useful sexual outlet for some people.

PENILE SPLINTS: These are made in various shapes, colors, and sizes and enclose the penis to a greater or lesser extent in an attempt to allow a man to have intercourse without experiencing an erection. They are partially useful in cases where lack of erection does not respond to sex therapy.

VAGINAL BALLS: These are ping-pong sized balls made up of various materials usually bearing a six-inch cord. Women push them into the vagina and the suggestion is that sexual pleasure is obtained by the user as she walks about. We have never come across a woman who has found these devices in any way useful or exciting and we fancy they are merely a sex gimmick.

SPECIAL CONDOMS AND "FINGER TINGLERS": Fancifully shaped and colored condoms (not always reliable as contraceptives) and devices that look like elongated rubber thimbles from part of the sex shop's trading stock. Almost always they are a disappointment to the users and their partners.

PENILE RINGS: Sometimes these are referred to as "love rings". They are manufactured in various shapes and sizes and usually encompass the base of the penis and scrotum. Some sex therapists believe that they have a place in the management of impotence in men.

REJUVENTING TABLETS: There are various formulations, but there is no evidence that they have any beneficial effects.

"LEATHER GOODS": There is an incredible stock of leather, rubber or plastic goods catering for those whose tastes incline them towards sado-masochistic sex. Mostly they are relatively harmless, quaint, and kinky sex toys. (Sadism is deriving pleasure from inflicting pain or watching cruelty. Masochism is getting enjoyment from one's own pain or humiliation inflicted by another.)

Alcohol And Sex

Q. Does alcohol make people sexier?

Ans. Small quantities of alcohol make some people sexier. This is because alcohol is a tranquillizer and tends also to release feelings that inhibit us doing new or worrying things. A glass or two of beer or wine will often act in this way. If more and more alcohol is taken the more it takes us along a path that leads us to sleep and oblivion-indeed alcohol was the first anesthetic used by doctors to put patients to sleep. A girl should know that an intoxicated sleepy person is in no way sexy, although she may be unkindly persuaded to have sex by an unscrupulous man, and a boy should remember the comment in macbeth on alcohol: "It provokes the desire but it takes away the performance".

Erotic Zone

Q. What is meant by an erogenous zone?

Ans. The erogenous zones are particular areas of the body, which are very sensitive for sexual arousal. Stimulation of these zones by touching, kissing, licking, or rubbing adds further to heightening sexual pleasure. These areas are very variable and what may be arousing to one person may be a turn-off to another. Sexologists talk about PRIMARY EROGENOUS ZONES, meaning the penis (and possibly the scrotum) in men and in women, the skin over the pubic bone and the lips around the vaginal opening to around the anus (back passage). They also recognize the lips and mouth, the back and sides of the neck, the ears, the inner surfaces of the thighs, the breasts and nipples, the buttocks and small of back as SECONDARY EROGENOUS ZONES. These zones are really very variable. Some people find having their toes gently stroked very erotic. Others may go wild if the inside surfaces of the fingers are kissed or licked.

Some Terms Explained

Q. Can you explain the terms heterosexual, homosexual, lesbian and bi-sexual?

Ans. Heterosexual means relating (sexually) to the opposite sex. A person is described as a homosexual or "gay" when their sexual desires and activities are directed entirely towards an individual of the same sex as themselves. A female homosexual is called a lesbian. Bisexual describes a person who is willing to have a sexual relationship with either a man or a woman. (Sometimes called AC/DC).

Gay

Q. How do I know if I am gay?

Ans. It is not always easy. Studies suggest that nearly 40 men in every 100 have at least one homosexual experience between adolescence and old age one man in 10 behaves homosexually for at least 10 years between the ages of 16 to 55. It also seems likely that 18% of all men have as much homosexual as heterosexual experience during their whole life. (They are bisexuals). The figures are more difficult to come by for lesbians but it is thought that 4% of people are exclusively homosexual and this includes women. They alone have no doubts about being gay.

Frequency of Sex

Q. How often do people who live together have sex?

Ans. It varies with age and appetite. There are few statistics but recently paired lovers may feel they need sex every day or even more frequently. In one survey of women in the mid 20s who had been living with their spouses for about three years, it was shown that they preferred frequency of sex between three and five times weekly. As couples move into middle age and over, the frequency drops to about once a week. Like everything else in sexual behaviors different people have different habits and desires.

Sex in One Night

Q. Can one have sex more than once a night?

Ans. Yes, indeed one can, but the reactions and sexual needs of both partners are involved. Theoretically women's sexual capability is unlimited from the purely physical point of view. In practice diminished sexual desire occurs after rewarding sex and although she can be re-aroused and indeed experience (quite rarely) multiple orgasms, it usually limits her activity. Men have an extra inhibition in that after they have ejaculated (climaxed) they lose their erection and a period of time must pass before another erection can occur. This is called the refractory or resting period. It varies from a very few minutes in a very young man in a relatively new and exciting situation to a period of hours in the more mature man enjoying a more long standing relationship.

Contraception Information

Q. Where can I get information about contraception? Does it matter that I am not married?

Ans. Information on all aspects of contraception is available to all men and women irrespective of marital status from the family doctor, and the family planning clinics.

Pregnancy during First Sex

Q. Is it true that you never get pregnant the first time you have sex?

Ans. No, this is not true. You can get pregnant just as easily the first time you have sex as on any subsequent occasion.

Groaning and Shouting during Intercourse

Q. Is it normal to make groaning and other noises during a climax? Won't this be rather embarrassing if it is heard by other people?

Ans. Yes, shouts and groans do occur during an orgasm (climax). Yes, it can be embarrassing if other people can hear it (to them too!) and this particular lack of privacy spoils many personal relationships, especially for newly weds living with in-laws.

Non-Orgasmic Sex

Q. Is it unhealthy to have sex without having a climax?

Ans. No, it has no effect on physical health but some people find it very unsatisfactory and this may destroy their sexual relationship, particularly if one partner remains feeling sexually unfulfilled. Really this is a very variable subject and some men and women find non-orgasmic sex very satisfactory and pleasurable.

Fate of Semen In Celibacy

Q. If a man doesn't have sex very often what happens to all that semen inside him?

Ans. In young men who do not masturbate or have sex there is usually a loss of semen during wet dreams. In fact semen is produced on demand rather than by a steady supply. If none is released the manufacturing process shuts down. It does not build up inside and make a man ill. Contrary too much popular belief the celibate state (going without sex) is quite healthy.

Nymphomania

Q. What is a nymphomaniac?

Ans. A nymphomaniac is a woman who very frequently involves herself in sexual acts and repeated intercourse with new sexual partners. Men of course do the same thing but have not earned a medical term as a result of this activity.

Wet Dreams in Married Life

Q. Does a man still have wet dreams when he is having regular sexual intercourse?

Ans. Not usually.

Meaning of Period

Q. If a girl says that she's "having a period", what does she actually mean?

Ans. It means she is menstruating. She may call it "the curse" or "the monthlies" or "feeling poorly". Usually girls pass blood from the vagina for four to five days every 28 days. This is a menstrual period.

Four Lips Down Below

Q. Do all girls and women have two large and two small "lips" down below?

Ans. Yes there are four lips down there, as you have described. The outer (larger) ones are called labia majora-the inner ones that lie inside them are the labia minora.

Coitus Interruptus

Q. Is it possible to get pregnant if a man withdraws at the last minute?

Ans. Yes, and the medical term for this is coitus interruptus -or Interrupted intercourse. There are two reasons why this sort of activity can result in pregnancy. First of all a small bead of fluid leaves the tip of a man's erect penis as sexual stimulation occurs. This often contains live and active sperm, which may enter the vagina and thus cause pregnancy without him experiencing ejaculation and orgasm. Much more likely, however, sperm is ejaculated without the man being aware that he is just approaching orgasm and the moment of ejaculation. Basically sexual intercourse was designed by nature with pregnancy in mind! From both partners' point of view coitus interruptus is emotionally unsatisfactory and may sow the seed of sexual problems in the future. Case studies of premature ejaculation and lack of sexual drive and orgasm in both sexes often reveal the past practice of coitus interruptus.

Clitoris

Q. What exactly is the clitoris?

Ans. The clitoris is a small sexually senstitive bump-a sort of female equivalent of the masculine penis, made up of tissues that fill with blood during sexual excitement. This makes the clitoris enlarge slightly and become slightly hard to the touch. The clitoris is located where the labia majora fuse and meet in the front. It is well supplied by nerves and its function is to receive and transmit sexual pleasure in the female.

Sex during Periods

Q. Is it all right to have sex during my period?

Ans. Yes, there is no medical reasons against it. Some religions actually forbid it and some people find it a bit messy. Again, it's personal preference that counts.

Sore Vagina after Sex

Q. After a lot of sex my vagina feels sore. Is that normal?

Ans. Yes, this can occur especially if you have not experienced sufficient lubrication during intercourse.

Unequal Breasts

Q. I am embarrassed at the thought of taking my clothes off for sex, as one of my breasts is larger than the other. Is this normal?

Ans. Most women find the shedding off their clothes embarrassing in front of a new person but with a loved person this feeling soon passes away. Breasts are very rarely symmetrical and it is common for one to be larger than the other. This normal anatomical happening is best ignored and forgotten about. You are likely to notice it yourself much more than anyone else would.

Pubic Hair

Q. Can you settle an argument? Is it right to shave off your pubic and under arm hair?

Ans. It is entirely up to you-if you do and don't like it, than you can let it grow back to normal again. It really is a matter of personal preference.

Virginity and Tampons

Q. I have been using tampons for some time now. Does this mean I am no longer a virgin?

Ans. The state of virginity depends on whether or not you have experienced (penile) sexual intercourse and is nothing to do with anything else.

Pain on Loosing Hymen

Q. Does it hurt when the hymen is broken?

Ans. Yes but not much and it is over almost immediately. Some girls especially those who have used tampons are even unaware of the hymen being broken.

Swallowing Semen

Q. If some semen is swallowed during oral sex, can it make one pregnant?

Ans. No, and neither will it harm one any way.

Meaning of Period 178
Menopause Symptoms 56
Menses and Virginity 104
Minimum Size 152
Morning Erections 126
Most Fertile Days 160

N

Non-Orgasmic Sex 177
Nymphomania 15, 177

O

Obstructed Tubes 142
"Old Wives' Tales" 146
One Testicle 121
Oral Sex 7, 168
Oral Sex Normal? 53
Oral-Genital Contacts 6
Orgasm and Nipples 94
Origin of Sperm 159
Ovarian Removal 138
Ovarian Tumors 123
Ovulation Pain 60

P

Pain in testicles 90
Pain on Ejaculation 90
Pain on Loosing Hymen 181
Penetration Pain 59
Penile Curves 23
Penile Dimensions 135
Penile Injury 30
Penis Enlargers 139
Penis Length 4
Penis Lubrication 54
Penis Size 27
Peyronie's Disease 68
Pill and Breasts Cancer 100
Plucking Nipple Hair 35
Popular Positions 38
Possible Conception 150
Potency after Prostate Gland Removal 107
Pre-Coital Douche 136
Pre-Coital Muscus 143
Pregnancy and Menstruation 49
Pregnancy during Breastfeeding 97
Pregnancy during First Sex 176
Pregnancy Signs 150
Pregnant Virgin 156
Prolonging Relations 16
Prostatitis 137
Prostrate Gland 26
Pubic Hair 180
Pubic Hair Growth 134
Public Hair 23

Q

Quick Ejaculation 111, 122
Quick Ejaculation anc Circumcision 45

R

Rectal Itch 160
Regaining "Virginity" 56
Relaxed Vagina 2
Removal of Testicles 25
Repairing Enlarged Vagina 130
Replacing Organs 132
Retaining Semen 64
Retarding Climax 87
Retention of all Semen in the Vagina 88
Rh Blood Factor 71
Right Time to Become 79
Role of Pubic Hair 35

S

Safe Days 118
Sagging Breasts 96, 159
Scrotal Cysts 71
Self-Gratification 84, 108
Semen Absorption 126
Semen As A Laxative 82
Semen Odor 61
Seminal Fluid 64
Seven-inch Penis 164
Sex Aids 171
Sex and Mumps 103
Sex and Weakness 170

Sex Changes 66
Sex during Periods 179
Sex in One Night 175
Sex in Standing Position 170
Sex Techniques 60
Sexual Advances 166
Sexual Atheletes 163
Sexual Response 14
Short Frenulum 24
Simultaneous Orgasm 13
Size Concern 74
Small Lump in the Breast 101
Small Male Genital 85
Small Penis 62
Smegma Secretion 65
Some Terms Explained 174
Sore Vagina after Sex 180
Spermatorrhoea 145
Sperm count procedure 47
Spinal Injury 149
Sterility after Abortion 105
Sterilization 123
Sterilization Effects 134
Strengthening the Vagina 155
Stretch marks 54
Stretching the Penis 155
Superfluous Body Hair 77
Swallowing Semen 39, 181
Swollen Testicles 67

T

Testosterone and Older People 45
Tests of Detect Breast Cancer 101
The Cause of Single Baby in Humans 47
Tight Foreskin 24, 52, 102
Tight Prepuce 120
Trichomoniasis 131
Tube Operation 143

U

Unequal Breasts 32, 46, 95, 180
Unequal Level of Testicles 25
Unusual Semen Colour 151
Unwanted Hair 162
Urethral Blood 112

V

Vacuum devices and Penile Injury 49
Vaginal Depth 5
Vaginal Discharge 22
Vaginal Relaxation 1
Vaginal Sensation 86
Vaginal Tear 111
Varicocele 72
Varicose Veins 154
VD Anxiety 165
VD Transmission 109
Virginity 37, 69, 87, 115
Virginity and Tampons 181

W

Waning Potency 66
Warts on Scrotum 106
Weak Drive 82
Wedding Plans 139
Wet Dreams 169
Wet Dreams in Married Life 178
What is A Fetus? 83
Wife Lacks Passion 58
Worried about Bent Penis 161

Other Books by the Same Author

- Encyclopedia of Medicine and Surgery
- Sexual Debility and it's Treatment
- A book of Gynecology and Obstetrics
- Injection therapy
- Modern Diagnosis and Treatment
- Male Sexual Disorders and their treatment
- Overcoming Sexual Disorders and Sexuality Transmitted Diseases
- Short Essays on Sex

Books Translated by the Same Author

- Medical Instruments
- First Aid
- Food and Nutrition
- Churchill Living Stone's Pocket Medical Dictionary
- Handbook of Preventive and Social Medicine